WHERE ANGELS CONSPIRE

*"Chronicles of a **transformational** journey forged between Canberra and Delhi"*

BY VINEET AGGARWAL

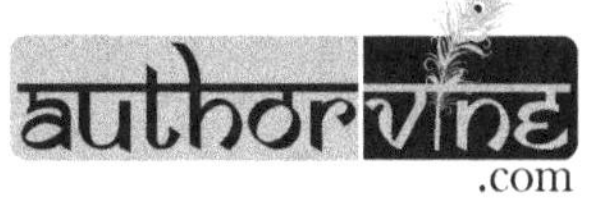

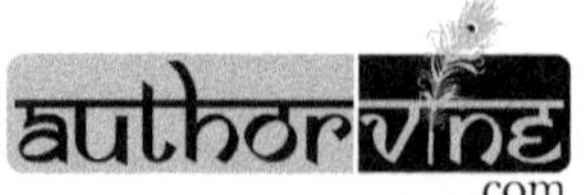

Website: www.authorvine.com
Email: contact@authorvine.com

First Published by Author Vine 2020
Copyright © Vineet Aggarwal
All Rights Reserved.

Title: Where Angels Conspire
Price: ₹ 499/- | $ 12.99
ISBN: 978-81-946060-6-2

"For my children Aviral and Ananya"

Chronicles of a journey which commenced with the mundane endeavour of losing bodyweight and transformed my life from existentialism to essence. A story experienced somewhere between Canberra and Delhi.

Do Angels exist, or is this just a word in the dictionary to describe the imagined characters in bedtime stories for children?

Let's find out.

Table of Content

Preface   i

1. The fine art of gaining 40 kgs   1

2. I am fat   45

3. Sounding the war bugle on my weight   62

4. The routine which caused a 36 kg Weight
   loss in 4 months   93

5. Oh my god, the weight is coming back   123

6. The billion-dollar heist around Weight loss   159

7. The window to the devine playfields   201

8. Reprogramming the subconscious to
   Shed some weight   215

9. Seeking some help from a little Buddha   258

End Note   279

PREFACE

I welcome you to this conversation between the two of us. For the next couple of hours we will share some of our deepest desires, the challenges we confront daily, the fears we live with, the heartbreaks and the problems associated with our ordinary lives, the feeling of being lost in this maze called life and the compulsions which force us to perform a dance which we sometimes don't enjoy or feel a part of.

By no means is this a one-way conversation. We will listen to each other's stories and find common ground as well as new perspectives to the same plot.

This is how we grow.

With individual experience, we grow one life at a time. With shared experiences, we build many lives in each life. It becomes bigger. It gets deeper. It finds meaning

From my side, I will share my experiences which have shaped my life and made me what I am today.

I was ordinary.

I still consider myself ordinary. What transpired that a

middle-aged and a middle-level executive in a multinational took this leap of faith to become a life coach?

I have no panacea that my story will change anyone's life. But I am sure that the experience which I am going to share will give everyone another shade of that ordinary.

When an ordinary gets a little better, I guess, it becomes extraordinary.

The period, about which I am going to speak, has had its own collection of hits and misses. Things which were extremely important to me at the start of that period became not so important by the end of it.

Something I was oblivious to became translucent.

Things I was enamoured with became redundant.

When I look back at the person I was, at the start of this period, I smile and want to have a coffee with him— a thought of having a coffee with my "that self" rings in a feeling of excitement.

But here it's about the two of us.

I am going to bring to the table my story, which started with a weight problem.

What changed in me?

What was the trigger to that change?

Who all were a party to that change?

How do I process the same thing now vis a vis at the start of this change?

As is the case with all of us, a story has characters; a story has its highs and lows, a story has some profound moments and events. Mine is no different. I will introduce you to some of them.

Was it just scripted and straightforward? Maybe yes. Or maybe no.

Were there moments of fear and hopelessness? Absolutely yes.

It's been a hell of a roller coaster ride and its replete with some unnerving moments. Some of those events still give me goosebumps. Those feelings remain embedded in my cellular memory. They are a part of me.

What unfolded, as an unnerving event at one point of time, became a nightmare in the interim and is just experience now.

This transition, over some time, was Something which I could not process at the start of the period I am alluding to. The one thing that has transformed is undoubtedly the "processing" of that period.

Is it the same as me?

Physiologically? Yes, except some ageing.

Consciously? Certainly not.

This conversation is not an autobiography nor some work of fiction. It has happened in real-time.

It remains like an insignificant speck of colour on the vast canvass of our combined consciousness. As trivial as it might be in its individuality but the colour is necessary to complete the canvass. There is a story in each one of us. Each story is a unique colour.

There was no colour like this before.

There will be nothing like this hereafter.

I will attempt, in the following couple of hours of this conversation, and spread between us the sheet of my life journey.

It has stains of those events which have shaped me. It has scars which have faded with time. It has folds which still unravel a new story. It has indentations of some folds which are now just memories. We will revisit them during this conversation.

I am sure that you will find resonance with some of those events.

Could be in totality. Could be with some variance.

If my reactions or responses to those events, can give you a perspective, which could give you some tools to process your own life, then this opportunity of having this conversation will provide a new meaning to our lives. The period which I will spread between us is from the year 2010 till the end of 2019. Nine years is a long period to live through when you are going through it moment by moment, hour by hour or day by day but just a flash now.

Nine years compressed to a few hours of this conversation.

I thank you for the time you are investing in me. It's the most precious gift one can have from anyone. This time will never come again.

It's in the "now", as we engage.

It is destined to be in the past, as we engage.

It will be in your memory.

It will be in my memory.

The same "time" that was just mine is about to become ours.

It will expand without any effort.

There will be two unique perspectives on the same event.

Where were the angels in this story? Do they exist?

The answer to those questions depends on the interpretations we give to events. Translations are the end product of processing.

That's how consciousness grows. That's how consciousness learns.

We are all unique expressions of the same combined consciousness.

I am so happy to meet a new interpretation of myself in you.

A self-called me. And a self-called you.

CHAPTER ONE

THE FINE ART OF GAINING 40 KILOGRAMS

I have chosen the year **2010** as a starting point for our conversation. Its relevance, to the context, will dawn on you as the conversation grows. You certainly must have heard the name **Canberra**.

Its a city in my beautiful country Australia. If you happen to be a non-Australian, I will excuse you for not knowing that **Canberra is the capital of Australia**. Most of the world has a notion that the Australian capital city is a toss between Sydney and Melbourne.

Don't worry. I was one of them before I migrated to Australia. That was about two decades ago.

Canberra has all the trappings of the megacities of Sydney and Melbourne. It is situated in between these two big cities. It has expansive malls, beautifully manicured lawns, lakes crisscrossing the suburbs, multi-cuisine eateries, a vibrant multiethnic community, some of the worlds best educational institutions and state of the art sporting facilities. The only place you will find one Australian icon. The Australian parliament.

The city, being the capital of one the most prosperous countries on the planet, is pampered regularly by the political elite of the country. So, by default, you are a recipient of the largesse and benevolence of the political elite who run the country.

Canberra was the city I called home, when we migrated to Australia, as a family.

The weather is most friendly for most of the year. Though, the winters are on the severe side. The community, being multiethnic, has so many shades to choose from. You can live a quiet life or a happening life or somewhere in between. The city has a well-spread buffet, for you, to choose from.

I was in a pretty decent job.

Decent organisation. Decent pay packet. Decent bosses.

Lots of "decent's", you must be thinking.

Life appeared to be well taken care of to anyone from the outside. After all, that is our full description of a decent living.

But was it as it appeared?

Or were there a layer of masks which I was wearing to camouflage the "ME" behind those masks.

It was diametrically opposite to what it appeared.

My marriage was breaking down.

To reach that point, where you feel that it's beyond bandaging anymore.

Where you get emotionally suffocated to the point of choking.

Where you are always in a state of anger and despair.

Where the word "home" loses its meaning, it just becomes an address to receive your postal mail. Nothing more.

This would be a rough description of my emotional state. Fragile and toxic.

I would keep working extra hours in my job so that I could spend less time at home, which had now become an address. I would drive painfully slow so that I covered the distance in a long time. Vehicles would zip past me. The drivers were sometimes honking, to express their disgust or anger or both. It was one of the tools in my emotional toolkit to shorten the emotional trauma which was waiting for me at home.

Many times I would just sit in some parking lot and wait for time to tick away. I knew the time my family would have gone to sleep.

There was school the next day for my children.

There was a job for my ex-wife.

Just before we proceed with this conversation, I would want to clarify Something in exact words.

NO ONE was responsible for my state.

Not my ex-wife. Not my children.

It's taken me a long time to process that period and share it with you with a different consciousness. The pain and trauma which, I was experiencing, was undoubtedly in any which ways not more than what my entire family experienced. All four of us were suffering the same pain. A marriage or any relationship just doesn't break up one fine morning. The point of break has in its wake a history of events. The location of the crack is merely an event which stands out like a sore thumb. Mine was no different.

It's just a reference point.

My physical health was no better.

I was almost obese, hypertensive, borderline diabetic and a whole lot of other ailments, which I could feel, were knocking hard on my body. My sleep patterns were majorly out of sync. I would get physically drained due to the long working hours, which I was loading onto myself to spend lesser time at home. And then my brain would keep me awake by weaving stories and conjuring situations. As a result, I would wake up in the morning with a toxic soup of my mental plaque. I remember consuming multiple serves of black coffee to bring in a semblance of alertness in my brain and some impulse in a sluggish body. I used to be in an absolute rush to make an exit from my home in the morning. Reversing my car from the driveway was the moment of liberation from a painful period of emotional toxicity and vacuum. A bruised psyche. A tired body.

There used to be partial healing of sorts when I got out of my house. Small things were my saviours. Some music of my liking while driving. Whiff of fresh coffee from my regular coffee shop. A nod or a smile from the same fellow coffee drinkers. No names were ever exchanged. But their presence was reassuring.

Then a mask would be adorned. A veil of a happy family man. A cover of being in control of my personal life. A mask of a fantastic evening spent at home.

Time used to behave so so strangely. I used to spend about nine hours in all at home. But it felt like an eternity. The fifteen hours spent outside of my home would get compressed into what felt like a brief period. It was difficult for me at that time to process why time was behaving so strangely. Though later on, through well-validated scientific and psychological explanations, I am much more equipped to decode this behaviour of time. It is this processing which I want to share with you. ***Something which took me nine years to arrive at, is here within your grasp, in a few short hours***.

Let's continue with my story. You must be seized of my emotional and physical state by now. There is a third state which completes me- My financial state. As mentioned earlier, I was in a well-paying job. The mortgage of the family home was being serviced. The children were in elite educational institutes. There was no shortage of any materialistic contraption for anyone. Between my ex-wife and myself, we were hardworking parents who were trying to give the best possible resources for our children.

The result was that I never had any significant savings.

"Why would I need savings?", was the constant logic I was reinforcing in myself. I used to derive priceless happiness in providing material things to my children.

The glitter in their eyes when they got what they desired. The so very animated conversations with them over the very inanimate objects. The discussions would transform the inanimate to the animate. I used to spend a short time with them during weekdays. Everyone in western societies would resonate with me on this. Weekdays are all about routines and schedules. A small part of the evenings and a significant portion of the weekends is about bonding and creating lifelong memories. I was no different. *Those memories are what I consume today to propel myself forward. In hindsight, I am so thankful to myself that I did not bother to create a financial safety net. That money would have got exhausted anyhow. But those animate memories are priceless.*

Those memories are a vital part of a lifelong emotional net. That net never leaves me.

But this realisation is all in hindsight.

In 2010, at that point, I was a toxic cocktail of a fragile mental state residing in a sick body and an extremely precarious personal financial state. And the most fantastic part of the situation was the well-choreographed precision with which the different states would feed off each other.

I knew eating junk food was not good for my body. But I was living off it.

I knew turning to alcohol would only exasperate my fragile emotional state. But it was my tool to escape.

My behaviour towards my colleagues was also nosediving. As a manager, there are certain expectations for your role in any organisation. And it was apparent to me that my tolerances with my colleagues were extremely low. I could observe signs of my judgement, failing me as regards my role. There was this creeping lack of ownership.

Everyone is bad. No one understands me. The world is all out to gang up on me. Why is life so unfair to me? Am I all alone in this world? Am I destined to this type of a wretched life?

This was the genre of my self conversation. This non-stop voice. This nonstop chatter. It was as if someone was sitting inside my head and chatting non stop with me.

Just due to my condition at home, I was becoming more of an introvert. Recluse, I suppose, is more apt.

I knew that I had this requirement to speak with someone. Just for venting out maybe. Or maybe just to get a perspective. But the fear of being judged was far higher than the requirement of seeking help. Even today, as we are conversing, the fear of being judged and being misunderstood is perhaps the biggest hurdle between an emotionally sick person and a happy person. Our society is not kind to individual situations. One person's misery is another person gossip. We invariably use chatter to hide our vulnerabilities and fears. We love speaking about someone else's suffering and then conjure up solutions based upon our conditioned judgement. This fear kept me away from any help. I had created this toxic cocoon to give myself a false feeling of safety and wellbeing. I was all broken up. But as long as it was not visible to anyone, but to myself, it was alright. I was conscious of the eventuality of my state. It was teetering towards self-annihilation.

Just to bring in a perspective, imagine you take a child to an amusement park and then abandon him. Just hide somewhere and observe that child.

The excitement of visiting the amusement park will transcend into fear. The attention, which was on the array of rides, will be drawn towards his safety. His eyes will only search for you. The smiles will give way to fear and hysteria.

I felt the same **metaphorically**.

The same beautiful city was not that beautiful anymore. The ex-pat dream of making it big in a foreign land was transcending into a fight to survive the mental storm.

The site of families enjoying bonding times in malls and parks used to amplify my despair and hopelessness.

The more despondent I got, the thicker the toxic shield would become.

My body and emotions were giving incessant signals of trauma.

Despair was my constant companion.

Memories were like the waves crashing onto the shores of my emotional beach. Each time a wave hit upon me, it took a piece of my sanity with it, a piece which would become a part of the depths of the ocean in front of me. The void left by that piece would become another wound on my emotional canvass" a wound which I would start covering up with the same toxic cocktail.

"Let yourself be drawn by the strange pull of what you love. It will never lead you astray."

RUMI

Why am I narrating in great details my emotional state?

The reason is that we create separations with each other by using colour, race, religion, ethnicities, regions and what not. But we remain *bonded with each other by feelings*. A feeling of sadness remains a feeling of sorrow. Its chemistry is mapped. We could feel sad due to any reason or situation. The chemical signature of sorrow remains the same. So are the various other feelings. Let it be anything. Happiness. Euphoria. Ecstasy. Anxiety. Depression. Name it. The chemical signature of every emotion is the same across the canvas. I want to utilise this bonding between us and give this conversation a mind and a body. The entire humanity operates in a narrow bandwidth of various emotions. The only difference is the way we process and respond to those feelings and emotions.

Everything we do in our lives is a sort of negotiation. We remain the chief protagonist all through our lives. The person or the situation on the other side of the table keeps changing. The result of any negotiation depends upon our responses to any given situation.

The small but unending sequence of negotiations is sometimes called life.

Any outcome, let it be as insignificant or trivial, will have a bearing on the issue of any future event. This connection will be explained and elaborated in subsequent moments of this conversation.

My life reached this moment one evening in Canberra, where it just snapped.

A small argument triggered the most significant upheaval of my life. I decided to walk out of my home. Just as I am sharing this with you, I can sense the same sensations in my body. Although way less in intensity. But their texture, their aroma and their flavour are the same. We sometimes have to live through such events and situations. There was no escape from these when they occurred. There are some memories which you wish to erase from your memory bank. But you can't. The only thing you can change is the way you process those memories.

Let me bring home a point. Imagine that you are trying your hand at a new recipe which you downloaded. You have followed all instructions and the processes to reach an outcome. Then finally you taste it. Let's say that it was a total failure. On eating the result, it will leave its memories in the form of taste, aroma and texture. Even twenty years down the line if you are made to taste the same outcome, even with your eyes closed, you will be transported to that moment when you had cooked that dish. Some experiences get entrenched in our cellular memories. I am alluding to those memories while sharing those events with you.

I did not have any place to go to that nite. Just my clothes shoved haphazardly in some shopping bags, a car, little money in my wallet and a badly bruised psyche. There was nowhere to go because this eventuality was never planned or factored in. The initial reaction was just anger. Anger gave way to fear in the next few moments. I clearly remember that I drove to a carpark and decided to sleep in my car. I was shivering with anger and fear. My entire life had crumbled in a matter of moments. And I was the reluctant witness to that.

I remember that I could hardly sleep that night. The discomfort of sleeping on the backseat along with the hormonal surge within my body was potent enough to keep me awake all night. A few short naps are all that I could manage.

The only question I was posing to myself was, **"now what?"**

I could barely wait for daybreak. Had to find a washroom and bathe. My primary body needs requiring to be addressed. They don't care if you have had the most challenging nite of your life. I decided to go to the gym, where I was a member. Needless to say that the reception was a bit surprised to have a member walk in much before the opening time. Just as a little note over here. I don't remember when my last visit was to that facility. All that mattered was that the membership was fully paid and it still had a few days to expire. Anyways. I used the facility and was ready to confront the next few hours. **This was when I had to start peeling off the masks which I had adorned**. There was no other way. There were not many options. I dialled my line manager pretty early in the morning. Usually, managers dread early morning calls from employees. And I was sure that my line manager would be extremely apprehensive about receiving a request at that hour from the person who had the keys to open the business premises.

On top of that, there was this shortage of words and vocabulary which could describe my situation and still hide my situation. I was just rocking between shame, hopelessness and fear at that moment. At the moment of my call being answered and post the first few words of pleasantries,

I simply said," I walked out of my home the last nite".

It was the first time since the events of the previous evening when I had **verbalised** the situation. And I verbalised it to an **outsider**. There was **shame** in doing so. But the question mark over my day to day existence was far more significant than that shame. I simply asked myself," how does it matter ?" My life took precedence over my embarrassment. What those words also did was that suddenly I felt a **load drop** from my shoulders. Metaphorically, *I had stripped myself of a mask*. Behind the mask was my **vulnerability**.

The conversation with my line manager was to the point and brief. There was no hint of **judgement** from the other side. On the contrary, I could sense **empathy**. The conversation was business-like, as I required a few days off from work to sort the situation I found myself in. The premises had to be opened, and the keys were with me. So my manager rushed to our workplace to take the keys. I was reassured that there would be no word about my situation with my team. However, the HR team will be duly informed. That's the protocol, and I was comfortable with that. Coffee with my manager post this long bruising nite was the best thing for me. I found that I had inadvertently rid myself of the **false male ego of invincibility**.

Another thing what my manager did was to organise an advance of my salary. I hardly had any liquid money at that time. And this single gesture went a long way in helping me find some ground to put my feet upon. I had taken four days worth of leave. Those days were spent in finding the cheapest possible long term accommodation. Working on some leads, I did find one. There was nothing like a choice in this. It was economical. And it was safe. These were the only criteria. It was like a hostel facility with common washrooms and kitchen. This would be home for me for the next few months. The place had independent rooms but other than that the facilities like the kitchen and washrooms were shared. So here I was in the most basic form of existence after chasing a dream of a good life for 43 years. ***It was a reality check***.

It was not designed as a men-only facility. But there were only men over here. Single men as myself. Broken men as myself. There were no pretensions. Each one of us had a story behind us. I remember my first nite in that dingy room. So many things, which we take for granted, in our daily lives, are luxuries you start craving for when they are taken away.

There must have been twenty of us in that facility. But there was no trace of any interaction between the residents. I could hear the sounds from the kitchen area at times. But neither did I find the desire to interact with anyone, nor was I ready to share my bruised emotions with anyone. I felt more relaxed after a couple of days, in my new frugal settings. A few customary greetings were unavoidable in the common areas.

I knew that I required to communicate. But I had shut all communication channels.

I knew I was in an **extremely dark place in my mind**. But I would not allow any sunlight to permeate those dark **recesses of my consciousness**.

The constant self-talk of being wronged, feeling hopeless, nothing to look forward to and being pulled by a mundane routine, we're starting to take me into a destructive nosedive.

I was living in a place out of my financial compulsions and doing a job out of existential constraints. At 43 years, how much worse can you perform in life? This is what I was telling myself.

And I was blaming everyone and everything around me for my situation.

I created a brand new bubble to insulate myself from the current situation. I would leave for work early in the morning and return in the evening and lock myself in my room. There was junk food, alcohol, television and my self talk to give me company.

But there was Something extraordinary which went missing. And that was the compulsion to maintain a false image of a perfect relationship. Everyone I knew, at that point, was aware that my marriage has broken down. There was pain inside me. There was this catalogue of beautiful memories. But there was no place for any denial or hiding this.

Denial is an extremely potent tool when it comes to dealing with any type of emotional trauma. It creates an artificial bubble of normalcy around frayed nerves. It helps one to maintain a mask for the world and yourself. We are always craving for validation for our actions. This craving for validation leads to activities which ultimately damage our consciousness. ***Denial is that mask which serves to achieve social validation***. My state of consciousness was no different. We might adorn a mask, but each mask has a weight associated with it. It's a weight which brings down our consciousness.

And all for what? Just social validations?

It is a huge price to pay for Something which doesn't serve us in any which ways. By the time we realise this fact, its typically post some **psychological damage**. Then post this realisation, we live with the scars. If we are fortunate, like me, we undo most of the cost and live normal healthy lives. But if we cross a certain **threshold**, like in many cases nowadays, then we are staring at severe lifelong issues such as **depression and other mental problems**. I was extremely close to that threshold. The most significant disease afflicting the entire humanity is not some form of cancer or cardiac issue. **It is mental health**. Some estimates put a figure of 60% of the adult population is or will experience some kind of psychological problems. I had a close brush with depression. The telltale signs were far too significant to be ignored.

I was deliberately isolating myself from any sort of social engagements or contacts. I would return to my living quarters in the evening and carry some fast food along so that I don't have to interact with anyone in the shared kitchen area. Consumption of alcohol had become a daily ritual. I would immerse myself in the mindless cacophony of the television just so that I was distracted from the noise of my self-talk. There were many weekends when I did not step out of my room from Friday evenings till Monday mornings except for when I had to use the washroom. No calls. No reading. No interactions with anyone. I could sense the degenerative effects of all of this on my health.

My breathing was getting heavier. I had started snoring heavily. I would feel exhausted and out of breath if I had to walk a few paces. Tying my shoelaces became a comic act. The layers of fat around my belly obstructed the movement of my arms towards my feet. The only way I could accomplish this seemingly mundane task of tying one's shoelaces was by lifting my feet, one at a time, on a chair and then reach out to do my shoelaces. My sweating increased exponentially. Even the slightest of physical tasks would drench my clothes. I was the least interested in any sort of self-grooming or being decently dressed. It used to be work clothes when at work and just two pairs of oversized track pants and the same number of 4xl shirts when at home. My bodyweight was galloping. The period which I am revisiting at the moment lasted for about two years. By the end of it, I had tipped the weighing scales at 123 kgs. All through this period, my routine did not change much.

It was the same each day. Pull me to work. Somehow log in the hours. Come back to my quarters. Eat junk food. Consume alcohol. Watch television. **And tell me a story life is good. That lie had become a part of my self-talk**. It was still toxic. I used to avoid shopping malls, parks and lakes altogether. Canberra is known for these. If you happen to visit Canberra sometime in the future, then you will appreciate the beauty of this city. But the same city was eating me up now. The sight of families sharing quality time in these parks and lakes would bring back my memories.

We are just a net aggregate of memories which we create in our lives. The events stay alive in the deep recesses

of our consciousness. Each memory remains anchored with some images. I will explain this in detail shortly. For me, the sight of these landmarks in Canberra would bring back the memories of my own family. Each park. Every shopping mall. Each lake. They were all a part of some image from the past a model which had some missing characters now. So I would bring them back from my memory bank. But I knew it was just a memory. Nothing more. This nothing was like the surgeon's knife. Each time my mind would conjure up, it felt that my consciousness being operated upon without sedation. My consciousness would scream. The only difference was that there was no sound. Only I could hear it. The only way I could insulate myself from that pain was to isolate myself.

Two words were my **protective shield, or so I thought. "Insulate and Isolate"**.

What I thought was protecting me was pulling me deeper and deeper into an abyss of self-annihilation. This is Something I realised later on in my journey of healing and Something which I will narrate in the course of this conversation.

Before I forget, a few moments back, I had said that memories remain anchored to images. These memories are also anchored to other senses like aroma, flavour and touch. But the most potent is imagery. So, for example, if I say the name, Obama. For 99.99% of the readers, an image will flash in their brains of the former president of the United Staes of America, though I have just said, Obama. Now there could be thousands, if not millions of people with that name. But for the majority of us, that name brings up only one image. This is what I was alluding to. Our memories are firmly anchored with images. I was consciously avoiding any such image which had the propensity of opening up my unhealed wounds. ***I was bandaging those wounds with primitive contraptions such as denial, isolation and self-pity.***

Why am I opening those wounds in front of you now?

Is it to garner some pity for me?

Or is it to grab your attention with a tragic story?

None of the above, my friend. I am just sharing those telltale signs of crossing the threshold. It could be happening to your friends, family and colleagues. It could be happening to you. This might help in identifying the signals. Something important that we need to understand here is that **sadness is not depression**. A person can't snap out of depression. Though in most cases, the starting point is sadness.

Sadness is a feeling attached to an event from the past. There is always a reason for someone to feel sad. Depression doesn't require memory to feel sad. You just feel sad all the time. Depression is a way your brain gets wired. It's a chemical and neurological choreography. This state requires trained professional help. It's not Something that can be fixed by the click of the fingers. Once a person crosses the threshold, which I have been repeating, there is a new chemical concoction in the brain to deal with. You can describe and mimic sadness. You can describe and mimic happiness. ***But You can't explain and mimic depression. You have to feel it. Your brain gets rewired.***

How do I explain to you this? Let me attempt. It's essential that we fully appreciate the role of professional help in this.

Say that I provide you with a fully paid course in flying. (I am just hoping that you are not a pilot.) The difference is that it is all online: no practical training or actual flying. The best instructors take you through the various nuances associated with the craft of flying. At the end of the online training, there would be an exam to test your knowledge and skills. (I know I am conversing with an extremely sharp mind). So you completed your online training and took the exam.

And lo behold. You topped the exam and broke all records of the previous scores. Your images are flashed on social media and newsprint. You are most well-trained pilot now.

Are you?

All your training and scores count to nothing when it comes to actual flying. You will undoubtedly be a total failure without the real exercise of flying.

Same is the case with depression. No one can understand how it feels because it can't be mimicked. It's a state of your brain circuitry. And it's associated with a chemical signature. Once a person crosses that threshold, beyond which the chemical soup changes, it's a very different ball game. There are so many cases of people having to live with that state. It's an incredibly lonely place to be. A depressed person processes an event very differently than a normal person.

There would be scores of people around, but you don't want to reach out.

There would be a constant heaviness in your heart.

Feelings of anger and grief would be your constant companions.

You would create barriers between yourself and the outer world.

Your sleeping patterns would be altered.

Your emotional state would become extremely fragile.

Family. Friends. Colleagues. Any sort of social connect loses its sheen.

There is this dark world inside your consciousness. This is where you want to be all the time.

So this entire commentary was simply to bring home a point of how we confuse between sadness and depression. The first person you need to watch out for is "yourself". If you encounter any of the above-mentioned traits in your personality, then reach out for professional help. If caught in time, it's completely reversible. It certainly is treatable. But if left to yourself or the ***social media-based quacks***, then it will only get worse. The world has lost immensely talented people like Robin Williams and Heath Ledger to depression. It is not worth a cent of your life to ignore it.

I was extremely close to the threshold line.

Maybe I was borderline depressive. I will elucidate this in our conversation. So hang on.

My emotional state had started expressing itself in my physicality as well. But I had blissfully ignored those signals.

My performance in my job had taken a hit. All my KPI's were in the red zone. People from corporate backgrounds would understand this. It's a cruel world out there. You have a job description, and there are numbers which define you. These numbers are called Key performance indicators. Or just KPI's in short. So everyone is chasing these numbers in the corporate world. My numbers are dependant upon the numbers of my team members numbers. My line managers numbers are dependant upon the numbers of people reporting to him, like myself. His bosses numbers are dependant upon the numbers of people like my line manager. It's a number game. The longevity of your job is dependant upon these numbers. There are periodic appraisal reviews of each person. If the business entity does well, again number based, at the end of a financial year, there could be bonuses for everyone, but again, depending upon your KPI's. Each employee looks forward to these bonuses. All for different reasons, though. Could be a holiday. Or a renovation in the family home. Or a new car. Or simple saving. **For me, it was just to save my job**. There was this constant fear of losing my job due to the low numbers of my KPI's. Somehow the numbers were just above the "firing line". The bonus was never my focus because I knew well how good or bad a job I was delivering.

There were these fleeting moments when I would question myself about my attitude towards my present state. Just a small quiet voice from the deep recesses of my consciousness. It was a very feeble voice. It was soft. It was loving. I would be drawn to it. **The cacophony around my consciousness was too loud and potent. That small, still and quiet voice would drown and get lost in that melee**. I could not understand or define that voice at that point in time in my life. There would be unanswered questions staring at my consciousness.

"If you want the truth, I'll tell you the truth: Listen to the secret sound, the real sound, which is inside you."

Saint KABIR

What do I want?

Is this the way the rest of my life is going to be?

Why and how did I reach this state in my life?

Am I so bad a person that no one wants to understand and help?

Is there a Devine curse on me to suffer like this?

There was an endless array of unanswered questions.

But there was one question which never came to me. And that was, **"What actions have I committed to being in this state ?"**

My friend, I am not going to attempt to judge anyone's situation. But if you are honest to yourself, Absolutely meaning absolutely objective, you will concur with me that our actions decide our outcomes. Each outcome is the starting point of another journey. Another negotiation. Remember we had discussed just a few moments ago that how everything in this world is a negotiation. **The only reason we don't ask ourselves the above question is that it has the potency of destroying our state of denial.**

And that's a scary proposition. We create a counter-narrative to justify our state of denial.

How can I allow anyone, even myself, to destroy the **ignorant bliss** associated with denial?

Why should the masks, which I am wearing, be peeled off?

Why should the world, myself included, be able to see my scars and wounds?

I was deliberately avoiding uncomfortable questions. I was oblivious to the fact that the starting point for the process of healing was myself. I was trying to disassociate myself from my state.

Does it feel convenient? Yes, it certainly appears to be.

Does it work? No.

Our life, its trajectory, its path, its milestones, its outcomes are all our responsibility. It's also called *"taking ownership"*. As long as we avoid taking ownership of our lives, we will continuously be grappling with the toxic soup of denial, self-pity and hopelessness. There is simply no escape from this. I was undoubtedly swimming or instead drowning in that toxic soup.

Remember the small soft voice I mentioned a short while ago. That voice wanted Something to change. But how?

That voice wanted help. But from where?

This is where my story took a huge turn. Nothing Devine or celestial. Maybe a fantastic coincidence. I will leave it to your judgement to give this incident a nomenclature. And kindly be patient in hearing me out.

The entire conversation, from hereafter, is anchored to this seemingly ordinary incident. But for me, this turned out to be the most profound incident for the trajectory of my life.

So here we go.

As mentioned earlier, I would consciously avoid visiting any shopping malls or public places. Nor was there a desire neither any need. It was a routine based on mere survival, nothing more and nothing less. My salary was enough to service my survival. Rent was a massive component of my expenses. Alcohol is expensive in Australia. Plus I had a mortgage on my fancy car which was bought, as an impulse, when I was still with my family. To cut a long story short. My money was apportioned accordingly. There was not much leeway to manoeuvre. To take care of all my expenses, I would continuously lookout for deals on fast food and consumables. One of the consumables was the trash bag which goes inside the vacuum cleaner. It gets filled after a couple of weeks and has to be replaced. I saw this deal being offered by one of the dealers in a mall. The first instinctive reaction was, "No. I am not going to a public place". But then I saw another deal being offered by a fast food outlet in the same mall. Now the calculator in my mind started working. I saw merit in making this short trip and save up a few dollars for myself to service Something else. So I chose a time when the malls are generally vacant. That time is invariably just when the malls open for business. I addressed my fears that early morning would be the most appropriate time to do this. I worked out a plan in my mind to its last details. Such as which parking would I use, where would I go first and so on and so forth.

It was a Saturday, and I started half an hour prior to the mall opening time. This was to facilitate a coffee on the way and some music as a company. I decided to park my car on the terrace of the shopping complex. The only reason for this was that the terrace is the last choice for people using the car parks. For me, that was the perfect spot. There are elevators from the terrace which take you to the stores, which are on the lower sections. I reached the parking lot and parked my car at a spot which faced the exit of a huge department store. Just to paint a picture here for your convenience, Canberra has some of the most massive shopping complexes in Australia. And this particular store, in front of which I had parked, is spread over three different levels. Each level is internally connected via escalators. The topmost level opens to the parking on the terrace. I hope my description has created an image for you.

I used the elevators on the terrace to reach the level where the shops of my interest were located. As expected, I was the first customer in the shop, offering the deal on vacuum bags. The visit lasted about three minutes. The salesperson tried to sell me other things, which I was not interested in, as there was no requirement of those in my frugal lifestyle. We exchanged greetings, and I moved onto the food court. The outlet offering a deal on some meals had just opened. I was in a hurry. The person on the cash register was a bit surprised. I was getting a meal for lunch packed when typically people have coffee. This took another ten minutes. I was the only customer in the food court.

There was this whiff of fresh coffee beans being ground in various cafes. It was sensuous and inviting.

There was this enticing aroma of fresh bread being baked.

The entire air was laced with different cuisines being prepared for the morning rush.

For everyone else, it was delicious food. For me, it was a deluge of memories anchored to those aromas. Remember how we discussed **memories being anchored to senses**? The smells were attached to memories. And each memory has an image attached to it.

I was not in a mood to spend an iota of extra time than what was required. One part of me was admonishing me for choosing to visit the shopping centre. But then I was explaining to that part of me that its done now and I would never do it again. ***It was that constant chatter between the two parts of the same "Me".***

It was done now. I said to myself.

But I had no inkling to what was about to unfold in front of me in the next few minutes. No, I did not run into someone. Nor was there an accident of any sorts endangering anyone's life. So just relax. We are not here to create fiction. But this one event changed the trajectory of my life. Let's keep going.

I had mentioned earlier that my clothes away from work used to be oversized track pants and oversized shirts. This was to hide my bulges and save some wasteful expenditure to purchase new clothes every two months. I had grown many sizes in this period. Plus with no social interactions of any sort, there was no need to spend money on clothes. That was way down on my priority list. Another small and innocuous thing worth mentioning here is that there was not a body size mirror in my living quarters. There was this small shaving mirror in the bathroom area. That would suffice for the rushed strokes of the shaving razor.

This might seem very trivial to you. And actually, it should be that way. ***But the point which I want you to***

know is that I had not seen myself, in a full-body mirror, for two years.

Now let's go back to the shopping mall.

I was still in the self-talk and rushed into this massive homewares store. My car was parked on the terrace, the way to which opened from the exit of this store. There was no customer at that hour in the store. There were a few salespersons who were getting some bits and pieces of their jobs done. Let me try to create an image of this store for you. It's spread on three levels. The ground level had the home furnishing, apparel and toys section. The next level is all about home appliances which are like a Disney World for grown-up men and women. There would be deals all the time to grab sales. The third level is exclusively dedicated to furniture. These are all big-ticket items.

The merchandising skills of the sales team are horned and tested here. The floors are expansive and extremely well merchandised. A lot of resources are spent by these chains of stores to attract customers and get the elusive sales. You know, it's all about numbers everywhere. Numbers define you. Your life, your relationships and your choices are all impacted by numbers. There is no going away from that fact. All the different levels in this store are connected via internal escalators. So you can very well imagine the size of this store. I had started my journey from the ground level of this store. And it would generally take about 5 minutes to reach the parking lot on the terrace. I was navigating the escalators to reach the top level. The journey from the ground level to the topmost level was again laced with memories. **The toys section was brutalising, saying the least.** I was watching the toys as the escalator was moving up. One part of the image was there. The other part was being recreated in my mind. This used to be a regular stop with my children. They would want to buy the entire toys section. I would negotiate for a deal with them. Some promises were made. A few targets were set. Some were achieved. A few will never be. Those conversations came alive from the depths of my memory banks. And with them, the agony and despair. But the escalator kept moving. As if **mimicking time.**

These memories vandalised my psyche. I had almost made a solemn promise to myself, never to expose myself to these memories again. It was perhaps the validation for the construction of that toxic bubble around me. Everything I had done to create that bubble seemed appropriate and logical. Surrounded by this self-talk, I reached the top level of the store. My escape from this misadventure was just a few moments away.

It would be fine soon, is what I thought.

How misplaced this analysis was about to explode in my face shortly.

All these furniture sections are extremely well merchandised. An extremely intrinsic tool, to make the shopping experience **wow,** is the use of massive mirrors. These mirrors are strategically installed to enhance the look of the store and the products on display. This store was no different. All the boundary walls were plastered with a continuous line of wall-sized mirrors. In a way, the entire peripheral walls are covered with mirrors. The use of mirrors multiplies the size of the store. It's just an optical illusion. But it appears fantastic. Whichever direction you turn your head, you will always see a product. Some as actual products and some as a reflection of the products. It's an amazing experience to visit the furniture sections. However, it is not conducive to the health of your wallet. Maximum sales in these sections are due to this feeling created by the optical illusion. It's called impulse buying. The job of the mirrors is to create that illusion.

I was moments away from my illusion being shattered.

I was visiting a store, like this one, after a pretty long time. Not that I was not aware of the floor set up, but my consciousness was tuned to a very dark frequency. And at that particular moment, the only task on my mind was to get to my car. My eyes were firmly placed on the steps of the escalator. I had my car keys in one hand and two shopping bags in the other hand. The escalator brought me to the top floor, and the exit was visible to me. It would have been a walk of about fifty metres. There was furniture displayed all over the store. Most of it was laid out to a theme. The real estate of these stores is costly. And all effort is used to maximise the floor usage. On any normal day, it's highly unlikely that you will just walk out of a section like this one. You might not make a purchase. But you don't want to miss the experience, the feel of the setups. My walk to the exit was not in a straight-line. There was some manoeuvring required to reach the door. I saw the exit and decided to take the left side of the store to achieve it. A salesperson greeted me with a warm smile, trying to engage me in a conversation which would translate into a sale. He was on my left side at a distance of about ten metres. His greetings had broken the chain of my self-talk. I intuitively turned my head towards him to return his greetings. I made his task easier or instead killed his endeavour of striking any further conversation by saying," Mate I am just using the exit to reach the parking lot". He left me alone. No dramas at all till now. Just as I was saying this to him, I saw someone at the far end of the store. It appeared that I knew this person. It was a fleeting vision, and I simply was not in a frame of mind to stop and see who it was. But the man seemed very familiar. I turned my head the other side to avoid his eyes because it seemed that we had made eye contact with each other. There was no desire in me to make a conversation.

Who was the person?

Why the hell did I make this plan of coming here?

But I thought he was too far away and started rushing towards the exit. The same furniture settings which appeared so beautiful just a moment ago now seemed to be a minefield for me to navigate. Just as I was grappling with these thoughts, I had turned my face slightly to the right side so that the person doesn't recognise me. To my utter horror, that same person was now looking straight into my eyes from the right direction.

How could this be?

How could someone be so nimble to traverse the entire floor, from left to right, in about two seconds?

As before I purposely turned my head away from the right side towards the exit, which was now a mere twenty metres away. One part of my brain was struggling to put a name on that image. The other one was just cursing me.

Who was it? Where have I met him? Why can't I put a name?

Too many "why's". But no answers to this self chat.

All of this description, which I have attempted to paint for you, is to bring you to a **watershed moment in my life**. Remember how we had discussed the case of Mr. Obama to explain that each memory is anchored to some senses. Just as a name brings in an image in our minds, an image stored in the memory will bring out a label attached to it. If you have met a person or if you have visited a place or if you have seen some person or any image on television, then you would also have a label associated with it. I am not speaking about someone you are meeting for the first time or random people whom we cross each day of our lives. In this case, I was struggling to put a label on this image. I was sure that I knew this man. All of this was racing in my mind at a million miles per second. It was too much for me to leave this mystery unsolved. I was just about ten steps from the exit. I decided to steal a glance. I turned my head partially towards the right and deliberately impeded my strides. I was just trying to squeeze in an excellent glimpse. I did that. I did manage to squeeze in a superb glance.

The mirrors, meant for creating an optical illusion, had just broken mine.

The image, which I was struggling to attach to a label, was none other but mine.

It was almost two years since I had seen my full body image. There was no customer at that hour in that section. **Time literally and metaphorically froze for me.** There it was. I was standing in front of me. An old and sick looking man. Sagging skin. Receding hairline. Grossly overweight. Sadness was written all over the face. It seemed that some-one had just put a tonne of external weight on my feet. I felt drained of any energy. My lips went dry.

I felt a bit dizzy. So I just collapsed into a lounge next to me. I was not in a state to cover the last few steps towards the exit. I kept on looking towards the mirrors. It was a blank look. **I did not have the tools to process this.**

The initial feeling was of utter horror and disgust.

All through my life, barring these the last few years, I had been an active sportsperson. I never participated for the sake of participation. It was always to reach some competitive level. With sports as an integral part of my life, a robust physique was a given. I never had to think about my physicality. A reasonable frame was achieved by default. And I used to take lots of pride in that. A compliment here or there does an excellent job to feed your ego. In a right way though. My family, my friends and colleagues, had always showered me with kind words on my excellent health. So my health was Something I used to take a lot of pride in. It was always central to my routines. Even after migrating to Australia, I used to be actively involved in some physical activity or the other. Remember the nite I slept in my car? I had used the washroom of a gym I was a member of. What I saw now was how I had destroyed Something I had nurtured all my life, except for the last two years and a bit. The image in front of me had just one word written on it. Only one label and it was not my name.

The word was "abuse".

I had abused myself to the extent that I couldn't recognise my image. That small, soft voice inside me was saying," it's your own doing Vineet". For the first time, I was able to recognise that voice. It was always **"The real me"**. And I was steadfastly suppressing it. I was not ready to listen to what it was trying to say. I had created this collage of masks around that real me. I was escaping my fears by impersonating as someone I wasn't. I was creating stories and tales for my consumption. My worries would feed off those stories. My state of denial would get validated with each story. If a story confirmed my self-denial, then it was a good story. If it didn't, then it was a conspiracy against me.

I kept on looking at myself from a distance. This was the first time I had confronted my fear. This was the first time when I was taking ownership of the situation I had brought myself to. I was trying to gather myself.

There was anger. But not towards anyone except with myself.

There was hurt. But not from anyone except myself.

There were so many events begging some for explanations. Not from anyone but myself.

The entire duration, of the above event, must have lasted for ten odd minutes. My chain of thoughts was interrupted by the greeting of another salesperson. He must have observed me in a deeply contemplative mood from a distance and probably seen that as an opportunity to engage me into a sales talk. I knew it was time to move out of that store.

I knew it was time to move on.

Just a few words on this expression of **"move on"**. It's one of the most loosely and liberally used phrases in today's world. Most of the times, it is construed as an expression of getting over some hurt and starting life again. I don't blame anyone for using this expression like that same way as people can't uncouple sadness and depression. Moving on doesn't, by any chance, means finding a new relationship or a new job or a new friendship, ***moving on means to move away from the consciousness level which caused that outcome.***

There is enough psychological and neurological evidence to prove that the same consciousness state will produce the same set of choices.

Same choices are supported by the same set of behaviours.

And the same set of behaviours and choices will result in the same outcomes.

I will explain in detail in the subsequent part of our conversation about this "move one" concept.

For me, that visit to the shopping mall to save a few dollars was life-changing and life-saving. I would realise this later. I did not have the tools, at that point of time, to process the event in any greater detail. All I understood at that time was that I had destroyed Something in which I always took pride. My health. This part of our conversation will be replete with details. The latter part will be about the actionable's. All of us find ourselves, at some point in time, in a space where we feel lost and scared. We try to search for answers and solutions to our problems in the open world. This happens because we have ended up giving control of our lives to social validations and norms. Taking ownership has become a rarity now.

I am right. I am the best. I know the most. I appear the best. I am the most intelligent. I am the most connected. I am the poorest. I am the victim.

This constant feeding of our ego's, based on the comparison, makes us feel the pressure at all times. There is an individual limit to take this pressure. When this pressure breaches a specific threshold, it becomes stress. We can use any number of fancy words or explanations. The underlying truth is that all **stress is linked with comparisons**. And all stress is external. I am alluding to mental stress here. My state was no different. I was using all the above-mentioned terms in my self conversation. It's relatively easy for me now, years after that period, to process the circumstances in an entirely novel way. But it was confusing and tricky to navigate the labyrinth of life at that point in my life. This thick layer of masks blocked my consciousness. There was no way to see any clarity or process my situation objectively.

The mirrors in the store had made the first cut through those layers of denial, self-pity, anger and hopelessness. And as they say, ***the first cut is the most painful***. I felt that pain in all its glory.

It was time to walk to my car. I reached back to my quarters in about twenty minutes. I thought it took just two minutes. I had lost sense of time while driving back. I was engrossed in a verbal duel within myself.

Have you ever experienced Something like this, when you lose track of time and space while you are engrossed in Something which obliterates any other thought?

There will be a significant chunk of our conversation devoted to this aspect of our consciousness, in subsequent moments. For now, the importance is just to mention my mental state. The description can wait for now. I sank in my chair with my image playing out in front of me. I was reliving the entire experience of those final few minutes spent on the top floor of that store.

I sunk my face in my hands.

There were no tears.

But I was crying.

I was mourning my demise.

For the very first time, I craved for some human connect. Someone, I could just vent out. Someone I could ask some questions. I missed my friends. I yearned for my siblings. I missed my children. For the very first time, I acknowledged the illusions I had created around myself. The denials I was living with, the toxic soup of thoughts which I was feeding on.

It seemed as if someone had pulled away the rug of lies from over me. And when the dust of lies finally settled down, there I was.

Exposed. Bruised. Vandalised. Scared. Helpless.

There was no one in the vicinity in whom I could confide.

An interesting notation will be about social media of that time. It was exploding, with people simply lapping it up. It provided the entire humanity with a tool to connect and express. The scale at which this was unfolding was astounding. Compared to now, the social media tools of 2010 can be safely called primitive. A platform at that time which was cutting edge is now obsolete. But it was an exciting time. Young, middle-aged, old, rich, not so rich, you name it. Everyone was getting hooked to it. I was not a big fan of these platforms. Be it Facebook or Whatsapp or LinkedIn or anything else. For me, the mobile phone was just to make calls or messages. I had cut off any means to connect with friends or family. I was a migrant, and most of my connects were India based. All through the years, I had cultivated and experienced some great relationships. My entire family was in India. Just to give you a thought to process before we proceed, "I had not been in touch with any of these relationships since the year 2005". I simply vanished. I did not share my email id or mobile number with anyone in India. And I did not let any meaningful friendships to develop in Australia. That's the degree of isolation I had created for myself. My self-talk used to be around **shame** and the fear of being judged.

How could I let anyone know that my marriage is failing? This was a shame.

How can anyone help me? This was the **trust deficit**.

It's my problem, and I have to fix it. This was the **male ego**.

So here I was in my self constructed isolation. It was dark. I felt I was choking for life. I did not have any solution to my state. The accidental rendezvous with myself, courtesy the mirrors in that store, had exposed my fragile and toxic state to me.

The rest of that weekend was just spent coming to terms with reality. A reality, which I had been avoiding to confront. I was grappling with questions.

How do I start the process of changing my state?

Should I reach out for professional psychiatric help?

Should I connect with my old friends and family?

How to reverse this failing health?

I had no answers.

The moment of realisation about the state of my life had glued itself onto me. It was a new animal to deal with. A new dimension. A new challenge to negotiate.

I want to emphasise here that there was no sudden explanation to my state. It's taken me a few years to process that state and share with you the deluge of thoughts which had ambushed my psyche. Looking at it now, years after it occurred, it's easy for me to process that state. But when I was actually in that state, without the learnings I have now; it was like hell. There was no escaping from that horrible feeling of being absolutely alone and full of fear.

The only thing which was clear to me was that this could not continue and I have to seek help.

Enough of my state at that time. I am sure you must have got a drift of what I was feeling. The rest of our conversation will all about the process of dismantling the toxic web around me. The starting point of that journey,

Was it simple and straight forward?

Did I receive help?

Were there any life-changing decisions?

My friend, it's my story. And it's not fiction. Over the last six years and hundreds of seminars and workshops, I can assure you of one thing, the processing of my journey has helped over twenty thousand people. People have found tools to incorporate into their personal journeys. Those tools have just done one thing," They have shortened their periods of darkness and hopelessness ". Every life is unique. And every unique life has a unique story. The tools simply assist us in making the life of our choices.

I think we have made a great start. Let's order for some coffee.

"Half of your life is lost in charming others. The other Half is
lost going through the anxieties caused by others.
Leave this play; you have played enough "
RUMI.

"All human unhappiness comes from not facing reality squarely,
exactly as it is "
Buddha.

CHAPTER TWO

I AM FAT. WHEN A WORD STOPS BEING A PROFANITY AND BECOMES A FACT

These were the exact words which kept playing in my self-talk post that watershed moment. In the chaotic deluge of questions and no answers, it was only this thought which I could process.

Just to share a few statistics to medically define me at that time:

Weight 123 kgs

BP 175/105

Fasting sugar reading 110

Joint aches? Yes

Sleep apnea? Yes

Sleep quality? Poor

Height ? 6 feet or 1.81metres

BMI? > 37.

So here I am with a medical explanation of my health.

My BMI reading said that I was "obese".

I was also borderline diabetic and hypertensive.

These figures were arrived at a clinic where I went to get a medical checkup. I was chasing only a single thought in my mind. **"I AM FAT"** . Honestly speaking, that was the only thought I could capture and process. Suddenly I found myself ugly, unattractive and unworthy. Just keep a tab on the genre of my self-talk now, the focus had somewhat shifted from where it was just a few days before this. **It moved from self-pity to self-care.**

As is the case with most of the overweight people I wanted to shed those extra kilos, and I wanted this to happen fast. I started frequenting book stores to find men's health magazines and books on weight loss.

The sight of ripped shirtless men on the covers was incredibly daunting to handle. I would buy a magazine or a book and try to follow the various routines suggested. Being an Indian was another challenge.

The food choices were all western.

That was a big block. Or I thought so.

I did understand one thing though, my eating habits

were extremely unhealthy. Wrong to be precise. And I did not require a magazine to tell me that. But the denial I was in, blocked all such thoughts. Anyhow, with great difficulty, I started cooking a few meals for myself.

Just some. Not all. It was boring and repetitive.

I would still have junk food.

Now here's the funny part. I thought that if I slipped in some form of a physical component to my daily routine, then I could afford to have some my favourite junk food. You know, I was reading a lot of health magazines.

Time was not an issue with me to slip in a walk. So I started walking short distances to compensate my lust for junk food. A serve of junk food during the day would be without any guilt if I had done a short walk. **Just notice the self conversation. I was trying to get around guilt**. Because I knew what I was consuming was not correct, I would create this narrative around my behaviour of doing the right thing so that I could continue doing the wrong thing. (Please re-read this bit)

A short walk would give me the licence to consume a junk meal.

How many times have you felt like this?

All the literature I was rummaging through was screaming at me.

My food habits were atrocious. Let me share with

you my regular daily eating routine at that time.

I would wake up and have a mug of black coffee with at least three chocolate cookies.

I would get ready for work and collect a serve of cappuccino from my favourite cafe. This coffee would be consumed at my office desk.

I would go for a short break at about 10 a.m., with my line manager, and have another coffee. This time the coffee had a companion, A freshly made cinnamon muffin.

We would break for lunch at about 1230 p.m., and I would be armed with flyers of various eateries offering deals. My favourite was a burger joint, and I would order a big meat burger. (It was bloody tasty.)

We would have another short break around 330 p.m. for a round of coffee or tea. This would be from the dispensing machine in the office.

I would finish work by around 430 p.m., and on my way back, I would collect some fast food. A lot of eateries offer discounts at the end of the day to get rid of the leftover preparations. It used to be a good bargain for me and save me the trouble to cook anything.

By the time I reached my quarters, it would be around 5 p.m.

I would switch on the television and shuffle through the channels aimlessly. Around 7 p.m. I would fix a drink for myself. Most of the times it was some cheap scotch. Sometimes red wine. The number of drinks would vary between two or three. Mostly two. The bargain meal would be consumed during this period. All of this happening while shuffling channels on the television.

The last thing would be a decent serve of my favourite flavour of ice cream.

10 p.m. was my cutoff time for a couple of reasons.

1. **I would be sufficiently intoxicated by then.**

2. **The news programs would be over.**

3. **My body would be exhausted by that time.**

4. **The next day was on the other side of my sleep.**

This routine was repeated without many variations. The only exception being the Friday and Saturday evenings. Those two evenings would extend close to midnight as there was no pressure to wake up early the next morning. The two drinks became three. The one big serve of ice cream became two big serves.

Trust me; **I am convulsing as I am narrating** this to you.

How can anyone ***not be unhealthy*** after following such a diet regime?

This is more of a statement and less of a question

that I am making now.

But at that time, it appeared absolutely normal and innocent to me. It was just food Something which I required to survive and derive some enjoyment.

Something which gave me pleasure and happiness. The reality that it was damaging me biologically was irrelevant. The sensation of relief while consuming that junk food or alcohol was Something which became my walking stick. It created an illusion, albeit a temporary one, of peace and tranquillity.

My internal chatter would get subdued. I would feel free from those negative thoughts of loss and misery. My attention would be totally on the toxic junk which I was consuming.

I would be planning for the next bubble of tranquillity, which was food, while I was consuming the present meal. The time I spent consuming food was that bubble of tranquillity. I would learn the science behind this behaviour later in my journey. And I will share that in detail with you.

Today a better part of the world is fighting a war against obesity. This one single health condition is intrinsically linked with a multitude of life-threatening medical conditions. And it just doesn't stop at the physical conditions. Obesity is now linked to a variety of mental and emotional states.

Let's get back to my food routine.

All the health literature was telling me that my eating habits needed to be upended if I had any desire to get my health back. I was not ignorant of this fact. For my entire life, barring these last two years and a bit, I was extremely cognizant of my diet. I knew how healthy food looked and tasted. But I had inadvertently reached a state of denial and as a result, this state of my health.

"If you genuinely want to change your life, you first must be willing to change your mind"

BUDDHA.

It should have been effortless and straightforward for someone like me to reverse this. Isn't it? But that was not the case as I was discovering.

If I knew the difference between the good and the bad, then what was stopping me from switching back to a proper diet? I just couldn't figure that out.

I would decide not to have a muffin with my coffee. But the aroma of the freshly made muffins would overcome that resolve of eating healthy.

I would firmly resolve, at least I thought so, not to consume alcohol. But as evening turned into a nite, and I would be drawn towards the bottle.

I would go to the local groceries and purchase fresh vegetables and other ingredients so that I could start preparing healthy meals for myself. Invariably most of those things would have to be thrown in the waste bin after a couple of days. Because it was not easy to make myself cook Something for myself.

I would succeed for short durations of time. Sometimes two or three days. Sometimes for a meal. But I would be steered right back into those toxic habits. I was losing my battle with myself. I had no clue what was happening. And each time I lost a fight, a sense of guilt would settle within me. That guilt would feed the feeling of self-degradation. You start calling yourself names.

Looser. Unworthy. Devoid of will power. Lack of motivation.

The genre of the self-talk remains toxic, and you feel that nothing is going to change. I remember telling myself, "if you can't improve something as simple as food, then how can you change anything else". The sound of such voices was getting louder by the day. My frustrations with my addictions of food and alcohol were rising with each passing day.

This went on for about two months. I had bought a digital weighing scale during this period. Whenever I thought that I had followed a good routine, for say two or three days, I would expectantly climb onto the scales. The weight never went down. In fact, a couple of times it was more than what I started with. 123 kgs.

It became amply clear to me that this beast was beyond me. The doctors had explicitly warned me about my health and about the not so distant repercussions.

The good thing about this phase was that my self-talk had sort of shifted from hurt and loss to frustrations around my failure to shed weight. I would be consumed by thoughts around losing weight and how unequipped I was to achieve it. The knowledge from these health magazines and other literature was not working.

Something was amiss. Something critical. Something which was more than just diets and routines.

I was pretty sure about that. Thoughts of getting professional health started coming to me. But I knew that enrolling for a gym and getting some help would cost a lot. My financial situation would not afford me that luxury. I had this rent as a constant. I had this car loan to service. Whatever was left was not enough to seek professional help. I had to do Something to create that extra source of income or borrow from someone or just forget about fixing my health.

None of the above was an option.

So would this be the end of my endeavour to fix my health and, by default, fix my life?

Would I be sucked in that toxic soup of thoughts from which I was so desperately trying to come out of?

I was grappling with the situation. I would make calculations and try to squeeze out some money by cutting down on what I was consuming. I would enact different scenarios in my mind to see the various possibilities. All of these possibilities were dependant on certain fixed boundaries. Those boundaries couldn't be breached. Let me explain.

My salary was fixed.

My rent was fixed.

My consumable cost was fixed.

My food cost was more or less fixed.

My job timings were fixed.

The incoming and outgoing were pretty much balanced.

I thought of taking up a second job to generate a small income. But whatever was available was clashing with my primary jobs timings.

What could I do?

I thought of shifting to some shared accommodation to save some money from the rent I was paying. That didn't work mostly because shared accommodations are with university students, nothing which could fit in a middle-aged introvert.

I had not cultivated any friendships from where I could seek any financial help.

Then what to do?

After trashing all the above permutations and combinations, the only thing left was my car. There was a sizeable loan on that which I was servicing each month. It was a significant sum by any standards. The vehicle was not bought with a backup plan of a failed relationship. It was bought with lots of love. There were innumerable memories associated with the car. It was just not a car for me. It was my escape capsule, where I would listen to my favourite songs. The driving pleasure associated with an advanced machine was immense. I enjoyed driving it. My children loved it. But that was the only option appearing in front of me. It was time to take another hard decision. It was time to prioritise.

In my mind, I decided that I really couldn't afford this type of luxury. So it's better to sell off the car. Pay the remainder of the loan through the sales. And then buy a very basic car. It's next to impossible to navigate Canberra without a vehicle. **So I readied myself for another cut into my emotional flesh**. There was no other way.

I called up the car agency from where I had bought the car and took an appointment for the coming weekend. I took the car on a long drive to savour the feel one last time. It was a very well maintained vehicle. I used to take a lot of care to keep it clean and serviced. But I needed to fix my health, and Something had to be given up for that. I reached the agency at the anointed hour and waited for my turn to speak to the loan manager. All through that time, the only thoughts which were running in my mind were those of the moment when I saw the car for the very first time, how the keys were handed over to me. The drive to the southern coast with my family. Lots and lots of memories. While I was in this state, the manager, a young thoroughbred Aussie, came out and welcomed me to his office. Exceptionally well dressed and well built.

What can we do for you, Vineet? He asked in his booming voice.

Without waiting for a moment, I said," I need to surrender the vehicle".

Oh. That's not good mate. What happened? He responded with all his attention towards me.

I have specific financial requirements, and it's getting impossible for me to service the loan and look after those commitments. I replied.

If you don't mind, can you share a bit more? He politely enquired.

His voice was very reassuring, so I told him very briefly as to what had transpired in the last couple of months.

He pulled out my account on his desktop and started having a look at the financial history of the loan. He must have spent about five minutes with that and asked me to excuse him for a few minutes. He left me in his room and probably went to the owner of the agency. He returned shortly and smiled at me and started.

Mr Vineet, I had a word with my boss, and we looked at your payment history.

I was just listening. I was mentally prepared to leave the vehicle. All I was interested was to find out about the amount which would be available to me after all deductions. I had to use this amount to buy a vehicle which would transport me within the city. Nothing more. He continued.

Your payment history is immaculate, and we are sorry to know about your situation. We have a small proposition for you. See if it can help.

He had attracted my attention now. Somewhere I could sense some solution. But didn't know what. He continued.

We can reschedule your loan amount with a small penalty.

My eyes lit up at the thought of a possibility of saving the memories associated with my car and also fix my health.

Please elaborate. I requested.

He printed out a document and started explaining the details. Cutting a long story short, I was being offered an extension period for my loan with a buffer period in between. What it meant was that my loan amount would be stretched over an extended period to reduce the monthly commitment and also three months of a loan moratorium.

My friend, it's impossible for me to describe how I felt at that moment. I had not only created some liquid money for servicing professional help to fix my health; I had saved a load of memories associated with the car. It brought a smile on my face instantly. It was not a smile which was fake or cosmetic. It was a smile which was the result of genuine happiness.

I thanked the manager and completed some paper-work. All of this took about half an hour. I was a bag of sadness when I entered the car agency. I was a blooming flower when I drove out. A small passage of time changed my total emotional chemistry.

I saw my plans taking shape, and with that, I saw the hope of getting my life back in my grip.

There was no time for any further delay in seeking professional help to fix my health. Some extra resources appeared from within my limited resources.

I never got to meet the person again at the car agency. I don't remember his name. But I can't forget him.

I had encountered my first angel to speak. We think that angels and fairies live in the figment of imaginations of young children. Adults are not supposed to believe in such trash. But for me, that person was nothing but an angel. He provided me with a solution which was beyond my capacity. ***This is what we are told as chil-***

dren, "Angels can do the impossible ".

He did not have any compulsion to give me an option.

I was not his friend. Nor was I related to him.

He did not owe me any favours. But I do owe him one.

That one act of kindness from the gentleman put wheels under my flat hopes. I was ready to roll now.

Now it was up to me as to how would I utilise this opportunity to fix my health and life.

Its only action from here on.

Let's roll.

LEARNINGS FROM THIS CONVERSATION.

All conversations give us some new learnings. So let me list out my learnings from these experiences.

1. Take ownership of your present state.

2. Acknowledge objectively the state in which you are.

3. Hiding from the reality of your situation will not change the fact. Confronting the truth will undoubtedly do so.

4. Never give up on a possibility which seems impossible.

5. Help appears from unknown corners.

6. Happiness, sadness, euphoria, despair are just a state of mind. Most of the times, these states appear and disappear seamlessly. There is no transition between the change.

7. Get your priorities right. Most of the times, our present realities are a direct result of our wrong priorities.

"Take up one idea. Make that one idea your life; dream of it; think of it; live on that idea. Let the brain, the body, the muscles, nerves, every part of your body fully aware of that idea, and just leave every other idea alone. This is the way to success, and this is the way great spiritual giants are produced."

SWAMI VIVEKANANDA

CHAPTER THREE

SOUNDING THE WAR BUGLE ON MY WEIGHT.

The remainder of the weekend was invested in research about the various fitness centres around the place I was living at that time. I had to factor in the time spent in commuting from my workplace to the facility, the cost involved for the membership and a few more bits and pieces like that. Remember you can plan and rehearse as many times as you wish. But once you are on stage, then the act has to unfold seamlessly. In my case, this was extremely important as I had just managed to create some resources to drive my pursuit of regaining my lost health. I, by no means, could afford experimenting.

I chose a facility called **CISAC, Canberra institute of sports and aquatic centre**. This facility was close to my house and was one of the best facilities available in Australia. Google the name, and you will be amazed to see the same. I also had an emotional connection to this place. I used to visit this place with my children for some fun sports. So I decided to visit this and enquire about the enrolment and various programs over there. The facility is spread over a vast area, and it has two levels. The ground level is where I used to come with my children. I had never visited the upper level. The main action used to there. So I reached the reception area and asked for some help to understand the cost etc. I was very warmly greeted and ushered to the upper level by a team member. Over here, I was introduced to the supervisor who first explained me in detail about the various forms of memberships available and then he took me around the entire facility. There were bodies of all shapes and sizes over there. I was confronted by bodies like the types I used to see on the health magazine covers, and then there were bodies of regular people we see in our daily lives. There were lots and lots of shapes with whom I could identify myself. There was one thing which was missing over there,

There was no shame on anyone's face, regardless of the body type. I lost the shame around my body in that very instant. The feeling was extremely liberating. There was this realisation that there are many people who are struggling with their bodies, and what it needs is guidance. Not shame.

The manager ran through all the membership options.

Before we proceed any further, let me briefly attempt to summarise the environment around fitness in Australia.

Australia is a massive country when it comes to the landmass. But it has a very small population. It's about 25 million now. The entire culture is geared around sporting activities. Sports and outdoor activities are an intrinsic part of Australian society. It's a massive and well-organised industry. There are many industries which are geared to service this inherent aspect of the culture. So be it sporting apparel or sporting footwear or sporting equipment, each and every element is highly competitive. If you are in Australia, then this aspect of the culture cannot be escaped. It's in your face all the time. Just due to this cultural aspect, you will notice that a country with a small population size dominates the sporting events around the world. Be it Olympics, world championships or regional competitions, Australian sportspersons are a force to reckon with. Even ordinary facilities are way above the standards of many countries. **CISAC** is an extraordinary facility. And if you want a professional from here to personally train you, then you need to have a deep pocket first. Then you should be very sure that you want to do this. I knew I had a "not so "deep pocket.

After understanding the various types of memberships available, I worked out that I had liquidity to serve personal training for just over two months.

Not a very long time if you see.

But I had to commit myself if I wanted any change in my situation. So I opted for a membership for six months. I didn't sign for any personal training, to begin with. Memberships are not that intimidating as far as the monthly charges are concerned. It's the personal training which costs a fortune. When I say a fortune then take it on its absolute face value. The unique thing in the membership, I took, was that it included a complete diet program and also had three complimentary personal training sessions embedded in it. A dietician was assigned the task to make a diet chart for me, and I was also given an exercise routine to follow. All of this must have taken about 2 hours. I knew that I had made the **second-best investment of my life** by enrolling in this facility.

(You must be wondering why second best. Hang on. You will know soon.)

I chose to work out in the evenings after work hours. I used to reach **CISAC** at about 530 p.m. every day. The facility used to be packed with members and the energy used to be sky-high. Being a premier facility one would not be surprised to see some national sporting personality training. The most common sight was of the rugby team of Canberra. **They are called the RAIDERS**. Fancy name. I could recognise the rugby players easily due to the investment of thousands of hours I had made in watching the television. The energy was infectious. I would really want to workout. My routine was very simple. Nothing major, I thought. It had a fifteen-minute walk on the treadmill at a speed of 5kms per hour and a flat gradient. The first time I climbed onto the treadmill and started walking, within 3 minutes, I had to step down. My mouth and throat went dry. My legs and feet were exploding with pain. My T-shirt got drenched. I knew straight away what I had signed into. The instructors had shown me some lite weight training drills. So I would try to follow them. It was painful. It was difficult. It looked impossible. My mind would be in that constant chatter about the steep road ahead. The first week was filled with excruciating body pain. I would simply drop into my bed when I returned home. I tried to eat according to the diet plan. It was difficult to sleep in that first week. My body would be in pain. I would wake up with pain if I tried turning sides while sleeping. But I persisted with it. I can safely say that I could follow about 25% of the exercise routine and about 50% of the diet routine in that first week.

Looks like a disaster when we see it now. But it was not when I process it now. Let's process this because it is of utmost importance to have learnings out of this if you are trying to lose weight or if you are a trainer.

I could follow 25% of a very lite and simple exercise routine. You can read this in two different ways.

I missed 75% of the routine. This Looks like a total failure.

Or

I reclaimed 25% of the time spent in destroying my health. That looks like a huge success.

Then look at the diet part now.

I could follow only 50% of the diet, even under guidance. Not good at all.

Or

I unfollowed 50% of the junk food diet. This looks like a winner.

It was the beginning of a process where I was trying to regain the lost territory of my health. It had to be incremental. And it had to be gradual. Even now, when I train people myself in this field, I emphasise on these two words. So please remember them.

Incremental
Gradual

Well, let's get back to **CISAC** now. I went five times to the faculty in that first week. There was enormous body pain, and I had to break up the week into two parts. That worked well, actually. In my second week, I was approached by a floor trainer. I was required to book my three complimentary personal training sessions which came with the membership. These sessions are not open-ended. They had to be exhausted within a particular time frame. Else they would go void. I promptly picked up three sessions in the proceeding week. You are not allowed to pick one specific trainer for these complimentary sessions. Your preferred timings are matched with the available trainers on that particular day. So I was allocated a trainer by the name of **Sebastian Jago**. I didn't know who the person was. The good thing was that it would be the same trainer for all the three sessions. His task was to train me on various machines and apparatus in the facility. This was to help me achieve my fitness goals and how to use the machines properly and minimise the risk of injury. An important lesson learnt in this journey was of injury management during training. In our misguided enthusiasm to achieve some goals, we end up jeopardising the goal itself by losing precious time due to injuries. These three sessions were to help me get used to a self-driven routine. I was so looking forward to that. First time in my life, I would experience personal training. I picked up the weekend for my first session and then the next two on alternate days after that. Evenings always suited me. I reached the reception area in time of my scheduled session and was just waiting for my trainer at the reception.

"Hi, Vineet. How are you doing today? ", I heard this voice from behind me.

I turned to look, and I saw a 6 feet 2 inches tall hunk of a man smiling at me with his right hand jutting out towards me.

Hi mate. I am Seb.

These are my first memories of Sebastian or Seb, as he was called.

I extended my right hand to receive one of the firmest handshakes of my life.

Seb had this constant smile on his face. He was in the trainer's outfit, so I could make out how well built he was. He appeared like one of those cover pictures of Australian models on the men's health magazines. It was almost a fan moment for me.

We exchanged pleasantries, and then Seb took me into

the meeting room.

Once seated, he just said," tell me about yourself, mate".

I being a person from sales and marketing backgrounds so I could talk a lot if required. In addition, I had this toxic soup bubbling inside me, which needed a vent to release some pressure.

I went on for at least half an hour. Seb was just taking brief notes all this while. Not once did he interrupt my flow or ask any personal questions. I told him whatever I felt comfortable with. I did share my personal situation in brief as I thought it was important for Seb to know my exact situation. Only then will he be able to guide me. Remember he was supposed to be with me for only three sessions. Once I was through my rant, Seb asked me to climb the weighing scales. He also wanted to take other dimensions such as waist size, arm size and chest size.

Only two measurements are vital for us in this conversation: my weight and my waist.

Weight was 123 kg plus. No surprises here.

The waist was 46 inches. Well, that's a big waist.

Why are these two figures essential?

These numbers were putting a numerical value on the poor state of my health and the dangerous territory I was meandering in.

My fight for the next six months was with these two

figures.

My focus had shifted from my emotional state to my physical state. And with the path I had taken now, I felt there was hope to fix my self.

Seb took me to the floor and made me go through a very lite simple routine, as mentioned in the initial routine given to me. He was taking notes all the while. He gentle voice would always be there as a reassurance.

If he thought that I was not getting the hang of a particular machine, then he would jump on and demonstrate.

If he thought a particular exercise was a bit too much for me, he would ask me to stop and scratch it on his sheet.

If he thought I was trying to impress him by lifting or pulling more than what he asked me to, he would shoot it down.

But he would keep explaining the science about each exercise. He would always talk about a **clean diet** and how to achieve it. The time spent with him was like an encyclopaedia being downloaded into my brain. Over a period of just three sessions, I knew everything wrong that I was doing with my food, water, sleep and workout. I knew why it was impossible to shed weight even when I was trying so hard. To Seb's credit, he trained me for these three sessions as if I was a longterm client. Not once did he try to sell his services to me. He was full of **compassion**. And compassion is what I required at that time. He is much younger to me. But in his presence, I always thought that

I was a child and a father figure is holding my hand. I felt secure with Seb. I knew he cared about me. Most importantly, I knew, he was cognizant of my mental and physical state. The three sessions went well, and I had decided midway through the week that it was Seb whom I wanted to be trained from. It had to be him.

We discussed this after my final session. It was a long and detailed talk. Seb walked me through the various pricing structures and what was expected of me in that. Money was a tiny part of that process. Once agreed upon, it was never discussed again. All the discussions were around the process and routines. It was suggested that I take three personal sessions with Seb per week and workout twice by myself. I insisted upon five individual sessions and two by myself. It took a while for me to make Seb agree to this.

What a beautiful learning I had from this chat. The difference in money between 3 and 5 sessions is a lot. That is all that a normal reaction would be. With Seb that was not the only point. He was more concerned more about my recovery post those sessions. He made me understand something profound. **LESS IS MORE SOMETIMES**. Of coarse the money involved was also one of his concerns as I had shared my financial capacities with him.

In the end, I won. A program was laid out for the first two weeks. In all, I had committed my resources with Seb for eight weeks.

"Your body is precious. It is your vehicle for awakening. Treat it with care "…. BUDDHA.

It was all go from here.

My relationship with Seb was always professional. He coached me on various subjects such as biomechanics, nutrition and routines. But what I learnt from him were some life lessons which I follow till date and deploy while I am coaching people.

Those lessons were of **compassion, active listening, simplifying and realistic.**

Let me elaborate.

When people are in some strife, their emotional states are a bit bruised. Compassion really helps them to heal. It lays down a road of trust between two people. This trust opens up communication channels. This communication helps in formulating a plan. When we work on a well thought out plan, our odds of achieving the desired result goes up exponentially.

Problem with a lot of coaches is that they don't listen to understand. They look only to reply. How many times have you come across a very accomplished teacher or a boss who are very ordinary when it comes to transferring their knowledge to us? What use is your knowledge if you can't make someone else understand it. You will never get a good result. A good coach or a teacher or a boss is that person who can establish a communication channel based on trust and planning.

Five days a week of personal training was a lot of physical effort. There was no hiding behind that. The sessions were staggered to give a break after three days. The duration of each session was 45 minutes. I would reach the venue much in advance and do the warmup routine myself. Seb would take over from there and destroy me for the next 45 minutes. He pushed me hard so that it hurt but not break me. He saw me suffer but with complete attention to the minutest signal of any injury.

His commentary would be something like this:

Common mate keep going. Nah, you are going too fast. Your elbow is not at right spot. Flex your abs mate. What did you eat, mate? Look at your posture, mate. You can do better. That's a lovely mate. Champ you are a machine. Take it easy. You are almost there.

His voice would not let me think of anything else. And I had experienced this in my complimentary sessions with him.

He would text me a few times during the day. They would be like:

How's the body feeling mate?

Drink water.

What did you make for lunch today?

See you on the floor mate.

How was dinner, mate?

I hope you are not being naughty.

Just innocent-looking text messages? Yes and no.

Seb knew my complete routine, and he kept me engaged with these texts just around mealtime. His texts here and there would keep my mind on my nutrition. It also gave me the confidence that my wellbeing is on his mind. This was extremely important for me.

That first week was bruising. I went for those five sessions. But by the end of the week, I had increased my workout duration to 75 minutes.

45 minutes with Seb and 30 minutes by myself.

The 30 minutes which I logged by myself were of pre and post-workout sessions of Seb. I used to get extremely tired by the end of it. But my sleep was better as my body was getting used to the aches and pains.

Exactly after seven days was the day for measurements. I was not expecting any loss of weight as I could not feel anything around the weight part. But overall, I was feeling much better. So I went into the office area on the training floor to take the measurements. Seb asked me to climb onto the scales. It was a digital one. When you climb the scale, it does not give you a reading immediately. It goes blank for about 3 seconds. Those 3 seconds seemed much longer than 3 seconds. I was looking straight ahead.

And Seb said," 119.7 kgs".

My first reaction was of total disbelief. My mouth was wide open. I looked down to confirm.

Yes, it was 119.7kgs. I had lost 4kgs of weight in one week.

It was just not the 4 kg weight loss. There were some gains, as well.

My self-belief came back. I saw hope and light now. **I felt like a winner** after a very long time. I wanted to embrace Seb. And I did.

What was Seb's response?

A pat on my back and the words, "let's hit the floor-mate".

I saw a sense of satisfaction in his eyes. We had registered a small victory as a team. It was small in numbers but huge in its impact. The sessions were never the same again. Seb kept on reinforcing in me the science of weight loss. He was explicit in no uncertain terms that this 4 kg loss was mostly loss of water which my body was holding due to my previous lifestyle. But now I had rocket fuel instead of standard fuel running in my system. My workouts became seven instead of 5 from the next week. I would do lots of cardio on the days I was by myself.

Walking on the treadmill slowly graduated to very lite jogging for short distances.

The number of reps with the weights increased. **My spare time** at home was spent in doing **research on nutrition and wellness**. My visits to the local grocery stores became longer in duration as I used to read labels and find options. The initial two months signed up with Seb became four months. The entire body language changed. I hardly watched television. I started reaching out to old school time friends. My relationship with my team members improved vastly.

By the end of 4 months, I was running on the treadmill at 9 km an hour for 1 hour nonstop. I was lifting heavyweights. The weight was falling off my body steadily. I remember the last weigh in with Seb. I had got stuck with a particular weight for about a week, and it was like the final hurdle. So Seb and I decided to give it a real hard push. We made an intense schedule for a period of 10 days. It was designed to be tough as we were chasing a tough target. We went through it. So we went in to take the weight, and both of us were anxious. I climbed the scales, and this time Seb laughed.

It came out at 87.2 kgs.

Both of us were laughing hysterically inside the room. I remember jumping in excitement.

I just couldn't believe this. *I had lost about 36 kgs of body weight in 4 months*. That is about 29 % of my previous weight. My waist size had become 34». Remember it was 46».

So let's lay this down again:

Weight down from 123 kgs to 87.2 kgs.

Waist down from 46 inches to 34 inches.

But was this all that I had lost? Think again. I lost much more than this.

- **I lost my fear.**
- **I lost my body shame.**
- **I lost my despair.**
- **I lost my isolation.**
- **I lost my toxic bubble.**
- **I lost all the misconceptions about health and nutrition.**
- **I lost my negative self-talk.**

And what did I gain by losing all these?

- **I gained sound sleep.**
- **I gained a new pivot, called health, around which my life Was circulating now.**
- **I attracted attention in the right way around myself.**
- **I gained recognition for what I had achieved by way of compliments.**
- **I gained reasons to be happy all the times.**
- **I gained new friends.**
- **I gained new opportunities.**
- **The biggest gain," I FOUND MEANING IN LIFE".**

I have trained in excess of 20000 people in the last five

years, virtual and live shows, by way of seminars, workshops, webinars and lectures. Irrespective of the audience and irrespective of the subject, the underlying bedrock of any endeavour is **"FINDING A PURPOSE TO DO IT".** Until you find a purpose to do something, it's next to impossible to get the desired results. It's taken me ten years to understand the mechanics of human psychology slightly. And I can state with a certain degree of confidence that

"it's the psychology of the person which controls the reality of that person. "

I will elaborate this in detail in the latter part of our conversation.

What changed inside me when I saw the scales after training for just a week with Seb?

I had lost only 4kgs in that 1st week. Not a significant number compared to the target weight.

My financial state was just as before.

My personal life was non-existent.

My health was still in perilous territory.

What changed was that I had found meaning, some purpose and some hope. It was a tiny click. But a critical one. **With one small click**, the state of my consciousness was diverted from

Negative self talk

Blame game

Hopelessness

Isolation

Bad self-image

To

Positive talk around a new pivot.

Ownership of my life.

Light at the end of the tunnel.

Acceptance of my state and the confidence that I can redeem it.

As promised earlier, I will state the **best investment I have made in life**. It was the investment in my own health by hiring Seb. I have come across scores of people who can't **differentiate between cost and investment**. Let›s get this clear here. The personal training that I was taking had a price to it. But that was an investment which I made for my health and wellbeing. I did end up paying Seb some dollars. But what I gained out of that spend is PRICELESS.

Till date, I undertake training in various aspects of wellness. Be it nutrition forms or yoga or mindfulness or sound therapy. It's always an investment which I make for myself. It is Not to make a financial gain as a starter but to improve my own health and gain more knowledge. If that knowledge helps me to grow as a professional and help people in a better way, then that's a bonus.

I had made the right decision of getting trained by Seb.

I am not in the business of astrology, but I can say with a lot of conviction that had I not taken that decision at that time, my life would have very different to what it is now.

"Become like the melting snow; wash off yourself; with love, your inner voice will find a tongue growing like a silent white lily in the heart "….RUMI.

Spending quality time with Seb trained me on so many aspects of communication. It was not a part of the job description, but I learnt the importance of remaining grounded, humble, patient, observant and realistic.

Let me give you a small example which stands out in my memory while I was training with Seb. Remember how I told you about Seb's appearance when I saw him for the very first time. He is solid and well built. And I was so fat and so weak when I started with him. But as is with most men, I was so enamoured by looking at some very fit people lifting heavyweights. One particular exercise is called the **"DEADLIFT"**. Somehow this exercise caught my fancy. It was part of the routine and was to be done on a specific day. The first time I tried this exercise, I spat froth from my mouth on lifting 60 kgs. The funny part is that I was requesting Seb to load at least 80 kgs. You know a big man lifting 60 kgs would look so feminine especially when a young woman on the adjacent station was repping with utmost ease with 80 kgs.

Seb just said, "let's start with 60 kgs and then we will increase".

Just after one set of 3 repetitions, I knew anything beyond that weight was not my cup of tea. Seb could notice the look of dejection on my face. In his inimitable style, he simply said one thing, "*mate never have an ego with weights. If you have an ego with weights, they will always feel heavy. But if you respect them, they will be your best friends*".

He then went on to demonstrate the correct way of doing a deadlift. I could see the strain on his body and his posture while doing it. He then said," 60 kgs is a lot of weight mate". He sounded genuine, and I found merit in the lesson about the ego part. He did not allow me to try anything fancy with that exercise that day. He knew I would do better. By the end of 4 months of training with Seb, I had executed a **DEADLIFT at 200 kgs** and a **LEG PRESS at 350 kgs.**

It was possible only due to Seb.

He had a plan, and he executed it patiently.

He was very observant of my progress. So he would increase the intensity gradually.

He always had a goal set for me which was just slightly beyond me. It would keep me interested, and I would achieve it.

He never boasted about his own capabilities and lifts. He would workout to demonstrate with the weights I was capable of.

These traits have become a part of my core now. I know it first hand how a person feels from inside when there is a mountain to climb in front of you. The last thing you want to be told at that time is your inadequacies. As such, when you are in an abyss, all you want is a hand which pulls you out. Seb taught me the art of active listening. I was never bombarded with lots of information or fancy onerous medical terms. The data was precise and simplified. It made the journey pleasurable. I used to look forward to my sessions with him. Yes, the workouts had become a pivot for my daily routines. But it was our conversation which was the most important. After each session, I used to feel that I have climbed out a bit from the hole I was in. Seb never took anything for granted while interacting with me. He made it sure that the concept goes into my core and becomes permanently lodged. And let me tell you, it's still there and thousands of people have benefitted with those skills, concepts and knowledge given to me by Seb. I always had the faith that my wellbeing is paramount for him. Even now, years since we trained together, his messages on social media platforms give me the same reassuring feeling. It's permanent.

As I mentioned earlier that social media was exploding around us. There was a lot of content available on health and wellness left, right and centre. For anyone who is facing any health or emotional issues, the material on social media becomes a magnet. I will not want to comment on the authenticity or the quality of the content, but most of it is feeding on human fears. There is some excellent content as well. But one has to very careful when searching for suggestions or solutions on social media.

Usually, the content is to grab your attention with titles such as:

1. Lose 10 kgs in one month.

2. ten best weight-loss diets.

3. If you have not tried this, then you have not done anything.

4. How this mom of 45 years lost 20 kgs without any exercise.

5. How this man made a million dollars in 1 year.

6. The morning routine that the Hollywood stars follow.

7. Get rid of such n such a disease by doing this or that.

8. Follow this and find the love of your life.

9. Do this and look 20 years younger.

10. How to become the best speaker in 7 days.

11. The best-kept secret of such n such bodybuilder.

12. Learn how this mom earns $10000 a month sitting at home.

13. Easy tricks to restore your boring sex life.

14. **Watch this before it is taken down by the government.**

15. **No gym wants you to know this weight loss secret.**

16. **The diet which is making nutritionist lose their jobs.**

17. **Say bye to your belly fat in 7 days.**

I can go on and on listing these out. Do you notice a pattern in all such opening lines?

1. They are trying to remind you of your **fears**.

2. They are telling you of your **failure**.

3. They promise **quick fixes**.

4. They are **flashing numbers** which will suck you in.

5. They will have **graphics** to make you start imagining.

6. They will make it appear very **easy**.

I was so lucky not to be sucked into this hogwash. I did try to follow some of this content in the first few weeks of my journey. But it was amply clear to me that all this information is:

1. **Generic at best.**

2. **Has little or no scientific base.**

3. **Has no genuine interest in your well being. It just wants to sell you a program or product.**

4. **Quick fixes don't work when it comes to your health and well being.**

5. **Someone is just trying to make a quick buck by stirring your fears.**

6. **It›s not at all safe.**

I followed these principles for myself, and I encourage all my clients and followers to follow the same. I remember a question asked by Seb to me in our meeting when we were working out a plan for my weight loss.

He asked," **what do you think is a realistic time for you to lose 40 kgs ?"**

That is how much overweight I was. My reply was," I don't know". He told me that it would take a minimum of a year off regular workouts and clean eating to get rid of that sort of weight by any average person who follows a simple but disciplined regime. I was not given any unrealistic time frame to suck me in a program. The conversation was honest, and it gave results. In subsequent years of my professional life, I have seen people do better than what I achieved. I have also seen people achieve reasonably good results. But I have also seen some totally disastrous results. They will all be discussed in the course of this discussion.

In a short span of 4 months, my life had turned around. The pivot was my physicality. But my psychology changed as well. Gone was the toxic self-talk. I was so much happier. I used to be smiling all the time. Work became fun. Feelings of being wronged disappeared. I was wearing good clothes again. I reconnected with so many of my mates in India. I started looking forward to a new start in my life. I started interacting with my children. My job was no more just a means for survival. I started feeling ambitious for my career again. I was opening up to the idea of getting into a new relationship. I used to go on long drives and enjoy the beautiful surroundings.

I WAS ALIVE AGAIN.

I was in love with myself. My body language changed from being resigned and lumbered to being enthusiastic and purposeful. Something extremely important changed. And that was my relationship with food.

Listen to this carefully. Food used to be some sort of a gastronomical and orgasmic escape from my drudgery. It was not like that any more.

FOOD = FUEL. Full stop.

I recognised that food had become an escape for me. With Seb, I started understanding the chemistry behind it. I started reading about food and nutrition as a man possessed. So many questions which seemed abstract before had now an answer and reasoning. Questions like:

Why can't I resist that if it's bad for me?

How can I gain so much weight if I have just a bit of that?

Why do I feel so hungry all the time?

I eat so much then why don't I have energy?

Why isn't the weight falling off?

Why am I not losing weight when I hardly eat now?

Why do I wake up so drained in the morning?

I am sure these questions will find resonance with anyone who is struggling to lose weight. For me, the meaning of food changed forever. It was fuel for my body, and it has the building blocks of my body. Now I understood the numbers associated with food. By no means do I want to trivialise your struggle with food. The lack of knowledge about food and nutrition is global. That lack of knowledge, coupled with our fears, has spawned a multi-billion dollar industry. And it is growing. I can lay a bet with anyone on one thing, that **If nutrition is made a top priority in our education systems around the world, it will wipe out 90% of the disease around the world in 5 years**.

Have you ever asked yourself a few questions like :

1. Why disease has increased so much in the last 100 years. Especially in the last 50 years.

2. Why just two generations ago, people lived a much healthier life.

3. When science has progressed so much, then dis-

ease should have gone down. The life expectancy has gone up, and so has the disease.

4. If fast food makes people sick, then why isn't a burger or a soft drink marked with a statutory warning like cigarettes.

5. If fast food is bad for everyone's health, then why is it allowed to be sold in schools where young children are exposed to those risks.

Remember I had mentioned about my readings when I visited a health clinic. I revisited that clinic after I had lost all that weight. You will be astounded to know that just in 4 months my blood sugar, blood pressure and haemoglobin count had become routine. All this without any medication. I was at an arm's length to go on drugs for all of these. And then I would have been on those medications for the rest of my life. So there would have been another sick person on medication and with a long life. Don't you see the connection here?

"Big Pharma. Food majors. Insurance companies. "

What a fantastic business model.

First, get them hooked to unhealthy food. Make their lives stressful. Let disease settle in. Make them cognizant of the dangers of ill health. Sell them insurance. Sell them health programs. Make them live longer but with the disease. Keep selling according to their fears.

I was a victim to this cycle. But not any more. My

health was my responsibility and the most crucial aspect of my life. Unless all of us make our heaths our own personal responsibility and understand that if our health gets compromised, then the quality of our lives gets compromised. Today we see hospitals teeming with people. There is enough scientific evidence to link most of those conditions to lifestyle choices. It's our utmost duty to equip ourselves with knowledge about nutrition and resolve that we remain healthy. When I say health, then I am alluding to both mental and physical health. Just like in my case, I could turn around my mental health by turning around my physical health. But I had to work on both of them simultaneously. There is no other way. You will understand this in far greater detail in the latter part of this conversation. The next part of our conversation will deal with some facts and figures, which helped me achieve what I did. But let's revise the few learnings I had from this phase of my journey.

LEARNINGS

1. Be open to new ideas. Never think you know everything. There is always something to Learn.

2. Be patient with yourself.

3. Start observing your self-talk.

4. Know your fears. Because your fears are wrapped in your vulnerabilities.

5. Revisit your relationship with food.

Keep this in mind:

- If something sounds extremely fantastic then most likely it's not true.
- Plan plan and plan. Time spent in planning will increase your odds of success.
- Communicate with people.
- There is no shame in seeking help.
- There is no shame in your body.
- Be extremely wary of social media content.
- Invest in yourself. This will be your best investment.
- Your wellbeing is your responsibility.
- Register small wins. They are easy to achieve and add up to big wins.
- Be realistic in your goal setting.
- Start slow and be incremental.
- Being humble and grounded changes your psychological chemistry.
- The mind and the body are linked. You can't fix one without the other.
- Simple is the best. Less is more.
- Stop looking for external validations. They have no value.
- It's safer to be with professionals than being with quacks.
- Know your weaknesses. Only then can you work on them.
- Erase self-denial.
- Stop comparing. You are unique. So is everybody else.
- Being overweight is **NOT A WAR.**

"Just as the water reflects the stars and the moon, the body reflects the mind and the soul"
RUMI.

"Paradise is not a place. It's a state of consciousness"

SRI CHINMOY

CHAPTER FOUR

THE ROUTINE WHICH CAUSED A 36 KGS WEIGHT LOSS IN 4 MONTHS

It's extremely important that I spread out the routine which caused this massive weight loss in me. I know you must be really inquisitive to know about the same. There must be a heap of questions racing through your mind right now.

What was I eating? How much was I eating? How many workouts was I doing? Was it simple? Was I consuming any weight-loss medicines?

I can very well understand that. I will walk you through the entire process and share with you everything that I learned from Seb and through the vast amount of health sites and papers. Many of the facts which I will share with you have been learnt in subsequent training in Australia and India. This knowledge has been refined over the last 7 years.

Let's start with some terms first. These will be used

throughout this part of our conversation.

BMI: BODY MASS INDEX.

It's a simple ratio with a formula as Weight in kgs/(height in metres square)

It gives us a number, and there are various charts readily available on the web, which will tell you what your BMI should be according to your age and gender.

Like in my case the number was 37. I was considered obese. I should have a BMI of less than 25 to be termed healthy according to BMI charts.

BMR: Basal metabolic rate.

This is again a number, and it is measured by a simple machine. These machines are available in any good gym or health clinic. This number tells you how many calories your body requires to function in an entire day with minimal physical activity.

In my case, it was 2260. This meant that I would require these many calories to cater to my essential body functions.

SIMPLE RULE: HIGH BMR, LOW BMI IS GOOD.

Now, what does this rule mean?

If I have a high BMR, then that means my body is burning a lot of calories to function. A lower BMI implies that either I am healthy or I have to lose lesser weight to be healthy.

So how did I gain so much weight in the first place?

The answer lies in another question.

What happens if I am eating more food than my body requirement according to the BMR reading.

ANSWER: remember my regular food routine of a few meat burgers, muffins, ice creams, alcohol, pizza etc. All of this added to about 3200 calories daily.

EXCESS CALORIES = CALORIE INTAKE - BMR

= 3000-2260

= 740 CALORIES (approximately)

These were the few calculations shown to me. (all figures are in kilocalories)

So what happens to these extra 740 calories.?

These calories are stored in the body.

Big deal?

Well yes. ***The excess calories are stored as FAT.***

Important note for you now.

EACH KILOGRAM OF FAT IS EQUIVALENT TO ABOUT 8000 CALORIES.

So the math becomes straightforward for my case:

I was about 40 kgs overweight.

40 KGS FAT = 320000 CALORIES. (THREE HUN-DRED AND TWENTY THOUSAND CALORIES)

These were a mountain of calories mate. Think of it this way, how many days of extra calories was I storing in my body?

EXTRA CALORIES / BMR

320000 / 2260

= 141.59 DAYS

My head starts spinning even now.

Understand the implications here. It's important for you to grasp this.

Theoretically speaking, if I did not eat anything for the next 141 days, then all this fat would be used to lose the excess weight. Our bodies use fat to store energy and use those reserves in times of lack of energy.

This is where the technical knowledge from Seb and other sources was helpful.

*****THE MAGIC MANTRA FOR WEIGHT LOSS****

CREATE A NEGATIVE CALORIE BALANCE IN YOUR BODY SO THAT THE BODY STARTS USING THESE STORED CALORIES TO KEEP FUNCTION-ING.

Sounds simple. Isn't it?

It is way more complicated than this.

An untrained eye would simply say that if I reduce my calorie intake by half, say by 1000 calories per day, then I would lose the weight in 320 days instead of 141 days.

Theoretically correct. But practically wrong.

Let me explain how.

Our body is the most complicated machine ever created. Modern science is just starting to understand bits and pieces of its functioning. The moment you start reducing the calorie intake drastically, I.e. less than 40% consistently, the body thinks that there is some food crisis. Hence it needs to slow down. Consider the following scenarios:

Scenario 1

Reduced food intake = body thinks there is a food crisis.

Food crisis = body slows down to reduce its energy requirement.

Slow down = slowing means a slow metabolism—results in a reduced BMR.

Reduced BMR = less calorie requirement; hence the purpose of less food intake is lost.

It will keep slowing down till it balances the BMR.

Hence weight loss will stop. I am not speaking about starvation here. You will lose weight from forced starvation. But there will be damage to your body. Our body gets all its nutrients through the food we eat. We need carbs, fats, proteins, minerals and trace elements. All of these are available in natural food. A right mix of natural foods will keep us healthy. The moment this balance is disturbed, we start suffering from various deficiencies. A strange fact which I learnt was:

MOST OVERWEIGHT PEOPLE ARE MALNOURISHED.

Excess weight doesn't always mean nutritionally sufficient. **Junk food has ZERO NUTRITION.** So when I ate a burger, I consumed close to 500 calories. But there is absolutely no nutrition in those calories. The body processes food to extract nutrition and energy from it. If the food we consume has low nutrition, the body again starts thinking that there is a shortage of food. Consider this now:

Scenario 2

High-calorie food but low on nutrition = Food crisis

Food crisis = Slow down

Slow down = Reduced BMR

Now compare the scenarios 1 and 2. There is a huge

qualitative difference between the two. In scenario 1, we consumed lesser calories, and hence the BMR went down. In scenario 2, we consumed more calories, but the BMR still went down. So in scenario 2, you will gain weight rapidly. As it's a double whammy. A reduced BMR will result in storage of the empty calories you had consumed.

You have to understand this delicate balance your body maintains. It's taken millions of years of evolution to reach where we are today. Your body is far more intelligent than the credit you give to it.

So what's the way forward then. Let's come back to my case.

What I totally understood was as following:

1. **I was 40 kgs overweight.**
2. **That translated to about 320000 calories.**
3. **I have to create a negative balance of these calories over a period of time to wipe out the excess calories.**
4. **Reducing my food intake below a certain point will be detrimental.**
5. **The nutritional component has to be maintained all through this else the double whammy will strike me.**

NOW THE SOLUTION.

A diet plan was made for me, which gave me about 1600 calories.

This created a deficit of around 650 calories.

An exercise plan was made which would require about 800 calories (this is what Seb thought)

That adds to 1450 calories per day.

Looked straightforward. But this was tricky.

1600 calories were not enough to keep the nutritional requirement of my body. Especially with a workout involving an 800 calorie burn, I would lose a lot of electrolytes due to sweating. Here is where the nutritional knowledge of professionals came handy. My diet was laced with items which were storehouses of nutrients. The food ensured that the nutritional requirements of my body remain fulfilled even with a deficit calorie intake. My BMR had to be maintained at a high number.

So these are the things I consumed within the 1600 calorie regime:

Seeds.
Nuts.
Herbs.
Raw nutrient-rich vegetables.
Egg whites.
Good fats.
Whole grains.
Chicken.
Fish.
Legumes.
Fresh fruits.

More important than this was:

WHAT WAS I NOT CONSUMING?

Processed carbs like white bread and white rice.
Soft drinks or packed juices.
Red meat.
Egg yolk.
Any sugary treat like my favourite muffins.
Refined cooking oils.
Packed snacks such as chips.
Alcohol.
Biscuits.

I will elaborate on my daily intake shortly—sort of a sample food routine which I followed on any given day.

Please note that all of this is what" I FOLLOWED". I am not recommending this to anyone. Simply because this was a very personalised program geared towards my goals and my physical condition of that time. This is just for your understanding as to how I reversed my atrocious physicality.

MY WORKOUT

This was the fun part. I used to train with Seb for 5 days a week, and I used to train for 2 days a week by myself. I chose to train in the evenings simply because I had to start early for work. There were strict instructions from Seb about my routines. I used to do a 15 minute warm-up. It consisted of some floor exercises and stretching. It was only after this training that I understood the real benefits of a warm-up. It's all about getting the heart rate up gradually and increase blood flow in the body. It minimises the risks of injury due to COLD STARTS so as to say. It was nothing fancy, but it was structured. Just in 15 minutes, my entire body would sweat, and I could feel the warmth in my muscles.

Benefits of a warm-up:

Increases blood flow in the body by gradually increasing the heart rate.

Reduces chances of injury due to cold start of muscle groups.

Increases the flexibility of the entire body.

Helps in raising the intensity of the workout.

It's a NON NEGOTIABLE.

I have noticed, so many times, people just don't bother about a warm-up. Needless to say, the results are not very encouraging. Injuries are common.

The next 45 minutes were with Seb, under his direct supervision. I would train a different set of muscle each day. Seb would show me the technique and explain to me the benefit of training that muscle. I started with very light weights. By the end of 4 months, I was doing some serious weights. They became my "friends". I learnt the right technique and body postures to get maximum results. There were some standard exercises. But every now and then Seb would introduce a variation. This kept the entire experience interesting and challenging at the same time. I use to have a lot of fun while training with Seb. My results had been noticed and appreciated by everyone there. Usually, it was the same set of people working out at particular times. By the end of 4 months, I had become a poster boy of weight loss. I really loved the adulation. But Seb kept me grounded all the times. All my routines were extremely structured. There was no room for any random routines. And the results were proof. My muscle strength improved. My lifts improved. I never had any injury. My recovery rate got higher.

Learnings from my workouts.

Structure it.

No ego with weights.

Posture is extremely important.

Recovery is vital to raise the level of your fitness.

Has to be a fun task.

Bring in variety with variations.

Sometimes less is more.

No room for random routines.

It is a common site in fitness centres of people simply gossiping and going through their unstructured routines.

If you are chasing some health and fitness goals, then your attitude on the floor of the gym will decide your result. I use to have fun. But it was never at the cost of my focus on the routine. Usually, it would be around my inadequacies. I would make creaking sounds to mimic the state of my body. And both of us would laugh. I was all the time cognizant of the fact that I had invested a lot of mine meagre resources to get something. I better not waste it.

Post my routine with Seb, I would be on my own for another 30 minutes. These were to do warm downs and some cardio. It was that little **EXTRA** which I was putting on this journey. I would jump onto a treadmill and run for 20 minutes. Then I would do simple floor exercises or just walk on the treadmill for 10 minutes to bring my heart rate down. By the end of these 90 minutes, my clothes would be drenched with my sweat. Just the feeling of doing a good workout was enough to keep me looking forward to the next one.

2 days of the week I was all by myself. Those 2 days were exclusively for cardio. My favourite was the treadmill. I used to be on the treadmill for 75 minutes. The entire session was again 90 minutes. There was no compromise on the warm-up part. Remember how difficult it was for me to even walk on the treadmill on my first day. By the end of 4 months, I could run non stop for the entire duration. In fact, by the year 2015, I was clocking 25 km in 3 hours on the treadmill. This 90-minute session is what gave me the edge. It was the extra effort which I was putting into this entire thing. When I started doing this,

it was not all hunky-dory. To even walk for 90 minutes was a mountain. I would amble. Then I would try to jog for a few seconds. Then I would walk again. But I kept on doing it. Gradually I could increase the jogging durations. Slowly I could increase the speed of walks. It was all gradual, and I had stopped competing with the invisible creations in my mind. I was seeking no validations from anyone. I was no more bothered if the person on the adjacent machine was running and I was crawling. That sight became inspirational. Earlier it used to be intimidating. ***These 2 days were the difference between losing 20 kgs in 4 months or 36 kgs in 4 months.***

When I started this routine, I would reach home absolutely destroyed physically. Within 4 months, even after a much intensive method as compared to the time I started, I would return refreshed and alert. I used to be tired. But it was a good tired.

In my later years, once I started training people, I kept all the lessons learnt in the period while I was struggling with my own weight. It sounds easy to lose 5 or 10 or 20 kgs on paper or as a commentary. ***The truth is that the weight goes down 1 gram at a time***. And if your knowledge about your body is not complete, then it's a difficult task.

I faced many challenges while on this journey.

Let me list out a few of them.

1. Cravings for my favourite foods like burgers, muffins, cookies, takeaway foods.

2. Alcohol.

3. Television.

4. Fried stuff.

5. Extreme fatigue.

6. Slow or no results.

7. Hunger.

8. Lack of knowledge about food.

9. Time management.

10. Social pressures.

"I give up freely what is no longer serving me. I release it to create space for what inspires me"
RUMI.

Let's take a look at all the above, one at a time. I am sure that you must be facing these issues time and again.

Understand one thing at the start.

"What we call an addiction now, used to be just a habit at one time". A habit repeated over a long period of time becomes an addiction. It is something which your body wants.

CRAVINGS ARE REMINDERS FROM YOUR BODY TO CONSUME THAT THING.

Your body keeps sending those reminders until the time you give that thing to the body. To break an addiction, you first have to understand the chemistry and circuitry behind it.

Let me take the case of alcohol. There is always a "first "time when we consume alcohol. It doesn't taste good. It doesn't smell good. Our first memories of the taste of alcohol are not pleasant. We consume it due to various reasons. It's possible that it's been consumed by elders at home or your friends have been consuming it. Let's not get into the social triggers for that over here. So you had your first few sips. The taste was horrible, and you asked yourself a question,

" How the hell anyone can enjoy this horrible thing".

It takes a few minutes, and you feel a bit lighter in your head. You can't process that feeling at that point. It just feels right. A few days later, an opportunity presents it-self again when you can consume alcohol. You know how horrible it tastes. But you also remember how it made you feel a bit lite headed. You talk yourself into trying it again. This time you consume a bit more than the previous time. You get the same bad taste and the feeling post that taste. Gradually you start looking for those opportunities to consume alcohol. **NOW YOU ARE NOT CHASING ALCOHOL. YOU ARE CHASING THAT FEELING WHICH YOU GET AFTER CONSUMING ALCOHOL.** It was the same story for me. I had never been a regular consumer of alcohol all my life. It was just social. But post my separation, I got hooked to alcohol. It used to make me lite headed and make me go to sleep. I was just chasing this. Same was the case when it came to having a muffin with coffee or a fried meal.

WE CHASE A FEELING. THAT CHASE IS TIED TO

A "THING". AND WE CALL IT ADDICTION.

I have heard, like a broken record, a million times the expressions such as:

I can't do without this.

My body needs coffee first thing in the morning.

I can't do without a sweet treat after my meals.

I can't resist the sight of that dish.

My body doesn't function if I don't consume this or that.

I have a sweet tooth.

I can't sleep if I don't have a little alcohol in the evening.

I can't do without rice at nite.

I can't stop eating when I see this dish.

This list can continue. I was telling the same stories to myself. And let me say you something here, "**ALL OF THESE ARE VALID REASONS**". This is your body sending signals to your brain, and your brain is converting those signals into your self-talk. I understood all of this, part from Seb and part from the vast amount of data I was going through and majorly through the science of **metacognition**. I learnt a few years later about this concept. It's a fascinating science, and I will explain more of this later in our conversation.

Coming back to the tools which I used to overcome my challenges as listed above.

The first thing I did was to write down my entire routine in a diary. I was absolutely honest in noting this down. It was something like this:

WAKE UP: washroom, coffee with cookies, another coffee with cookies.

BREAKFAST: 2 slices of white bread with margarine and 2 fried eggs

LEAVE FOR WORK: get a coffee on the way.

MORNING BREAK AT WORK: Another coffee with my favourite muffin.

LUNCH: grab a burger deal from some food joint

MID AFTERNOON BREAK: Another coffee with some cookies

ON THE WAY BACK: Grab some takeaway.

EVENING: 2 to 3 large drinks with some chips or fried salted peanuts.

DINNER: eat the takeaway.

SLEEP.

Trust me, I was on this routine with only slight variations over the weekends. It used to get worse on weekends. Now let's process this food (or should we say junk).

1. It has almost zero nutrition as there is no sight of

anything nutritious.

2. **It's loaded with BLANK CALORIES.**
3. **It's packed with processed sugar.**
4. **No one can remain healthy with this diet.**

So I was eating a lot of food, but it was working against me in all directions. It was giving myself a mountain of calories. And due to lack of nutrition in these foods, my

BMR was going down, and my BMI was going up.

Now is it making sense to you? I mentioned the golden rule sometime back:

FOR EFFECTIVE WEIGHT LOSS "LOW BMI. HIGH BMR"

And where was I?

"LOW BMR. HIGH BMI " = WEIGHT GAIN

There are many more contours to this. But I just want you to understand step by step as to how I managed my journey. This information was not available to me from anywhere. It took a lot of research on my part and help from Seb. My personal experience as an overweight person helped me to put a simplified version for the sake of our conversation.

This co-relation was vital for me to chart a path through the minefield of my addictions. There are some more facts which I would want you to know before we proceed.

- Lack **of water intake is mimicked by hunger**. Do you know that 70% plus of our body is water? And most of the times we misunderstand thirst with hunger. So I started keeping a water bottle with me all the time. I would ensure that I was drinking 3 bottles during the day. This was other than the water consumption in the gym.

- **More than 50% of food processing happens in the mouth.** I used to be on a sprint while eating food. As a result, almost all my food reached my stomach in a state where it would not be totally processed for the next stage. So what did I change? I would ensure that I masticate each bite in my mouth to a state that it was a semi-liquid. Then I used to gulp it down.

- **I started making meals for myself.** For this, I would invest a lot of time in the grocery stores during the weekend to research and then BUY ACCORDING TO THE WEEKLY PLAN. It's imperative that you plan ahead. Else you are staring at failure.

- **I stocked healthy options for snacking** so that my cravings are taken care of. These were seeds mixes, nuts etc.

- **I stopped watching television on reaching home after my workout.** Instead, I would spend time on the desktop to do research and also connect with friends and family.

- **My fridge, table drawer, car glove box, gym bag and office desk were all stocked with some healthy snacks.**

- **I maintained a daily** diary with my food intake and kept a watch on the calories consumed. There was nothing left to the imagination.

- **I changed my route** to work and back. (funny but it helped)

- **I stopped visiting the food court during my breaks.** Instead, I would go into some book store.

What did all the above achieve? Let's process that now.

* consuming lots of water kept me hydrated and helped in bringing my hunger down. I would feel fuller.

* chewing the food to a state of liquid would do two things. It made the food ready to be processed in my guts. As a result, my digestion became so much better. Secondly, it increased the time I was taking to finish a meal. Why is that important? I will keep it simple for you. There is a nerve in our stomach region which sends a signal to the brain that food is enough now. The brain then sends a message giving us a "feeling full ". So we feel that it's time to stop. **There is a catch here**. There is a **time lag of about 20 minutes** in this. And this is where a considerable problem hides for us. I would end up eating much more than my **REAL HUNGER.** So by taking more time in eating, there was a double gain for me. I was sending well-processed food to my guts and eating according to REAL HUNGER.

- Cooking for myself would ensure that my food was packed with nutrition, and it had the best ingredients. My primary goal was NUTRITION. The primary purpose of eateries is TASTE. There is a substantial qualitative difference between the two. Though let me guarantee you that the food cooked by myself was delicious and loaded with nutrition. It saved me a lot of money as well.

- By keeping myself well stocked with healthy options

saved me from grabbing unhealthy things such as cookies or chocolates. My snack was a seed and nuts mix which I used to make myself.

- Noting down my entire intake gave me a real-time check on my calorie consumption and my progress with quantities. I knew exactly what my numbers were in terms of calories and weight loss each week.

- By changing my route to work and back saved me the struggle of fighting my internal chatter of stopping and grabbing a coffee. It worked for me. Why? Later in the conversation.

- Going to a book store instead of the food court saved me from being ambushed by the aroma and site of the various treats being prepared over there. My senses were still a slave to these sensations. I didn't want to test them.

With these tools and constant training from Seb, I would negotiate my journey one day at a time. Progress made on every single day of those 4 months added up to a massive result.

There were many reasons which lined up and supported each other for my success. Let me list them out for you.

- » I wanted help and was very clear about it. This was beyond me. I had tried it for the first few weeks and would fail miserably because my knowledge was half-cooked at best.

- » only a trained person would be able to give this a structure. An unstructured approach is doomed for failure.

» I was sincere first to myself and then with my trainers.

» I knew it is going to take time. If I had taken a few years to reach this state of my health, then it was going to take time to reverse it. It's not a 2-hour movie in which the hero will become a world champion in 1 hour. I was ready for the long haul.

» I addressed all of my habits and routines which brought me to the present state.

» I equipped myself with knowledge about food, nutrition and my body so that I could erase the damage I had caused to it.

» I filled my spare time with activities such as reconnecting with family and friends. Earlier I would be glued to the television to "kill" time. Now I was utilising the same time to heal myself emotionally and decimate my seclusion.

» I acknowledged the fact that my personal life was in shambles, and I had to create a new experience.

"Most enjoyable activities are not natural; they demand an effort that initially one is reluctant to make. But once the interaction starts to provide feedback to the person's skills, it usually begins to be intrinsically rewarding."
MIHALY CSIKSZENTMIHALYI

I still use the same approach while training and coaching people in my role as a lifestyle and mind coach. The process remains the same till date. The only difference now is that I have a better understanding of the process now as compared to the time I was going through that trauma. There are many more contours to this. The more we invest in knowing about the mind-body connection, the better our understanding gets as regards the functioning of human beings. We all have been given the same 24 hours in a day. It's totally our choice as to how we use or abuse this time. I used to abuse these 24 hours by wallowing in sorrow and hurt. The same 24 hours are invested now in learning and sharing those learnings. There are millions of people struggling with issues similar to mine. I have been helping them by providing tools to redeem themselves.

Coming back to my journey now. You must have got a drift of my approach by now. All this would happen with clockwork precision. I would run through my notes with Seb and take his approval and further suggestions. I brought in variety in my meals. You will be amazed at what all you can create from fresh produce. My nutrition was vital because the calorie intake had to be on the lower side. So I would pack my meals with nutrient-dense ingredients. I became extremely watchful of my sleeping patterns, water intake, nutrition, recovery from workouts, posture and meal timings. I would grab the smallest possibility to work that little extra. Let me give you an example here.

I was a retail manager and had a large team to manage. What I used to do earlier was to spend most of my time in my office space. What I started doing now was just the opposite of that. I would spend almost all my time on the shop floor. And I would not stop in one place. Would just keep circling the floor. I was doing this to increase my physical activity and burn more calories. It certainly did that. But it did one more thing. Due to my continuous operation on the shop floor, there was much better discipline in the entire team, and that resulted in higher productivity. Remember how I had mentioned about the KPI's at the beginning of our conversation. This drove the KPI's through the roof. I ended up getting the much sort after bonuses.

So one affirmative action was a trigger to some other affirmative action. This energy feeds off itself. I was addressing my physical and emotional states together. The energy around me changed completely. I was happy to buy new clothes for myself. I would spend the weekends meeting people or going for a drive to the many scenic spots near Canberra. My favourite was Tuross Head on the southern coast. It's a 2-hour drive from Canberra, and I would drive and enjoy sitting on the beach. Reading became a habit. Making notes became a habit. I got ambitious about my career. I wanted to move forward.

The bottom line was that I wanted a permanent change and never be in the same space from where I had just escaped. **That one incident of mirrors was the trigger for change**. My physicality became the pivot around which I turned my mentality. That moment could have just passed by. But it didn't. My association with Seb was professional and remains the same till date. He was my coach and will remain my coach. He certainly is one of the angels who appeared from nowhere and helped me become what I am today… **Still ordinary, just a little better than yesterday**.

These 4 months changed the complete course of my life. I had this massive sense of achievement. There was a relief due to the demolition of the toxic bubble which I had surrounded myself with. The feeling was like when you are taken underwater by a huge wave, and you are trying to reach the surface of the ocean with no air left in your lungs. Finally, when you do succeed in breaking the ocean surface, the first thing you do is take this huge gasp of life-sustaining air. I felt exactly like that. There was this sense of liberation.

I have shared with you my weight loss routine with you. I have shared the coaching I took from Seb.

So is this the end of this conversation?

Should we greet each other and go our own different paths?

Have we accomplished what we set out for?

It is actually the beginning of a meaningful conversation from here on.

The reason I processed my weight loss journey for you is much more than some suggestions and processes about weight loss. What we have spoken till now is about the physical part of my weight loss. That is all about diets and routines. There are millions of routines available on the net.

Have you taken notice of a couple of things?

What I have narrated is not rocket science. Yes, it was personalised, but most of that information is available in public domains.

Then why losing weight is such a struggle?

Why do you lose it and then get it back?

Why some people succeed in losing weight and keep it away?

Why does a process work for one person but fails for another person?

What I will address in the remaining part of our conversation are these questions. It will not be complete if I don't share with you the **psychology of weight loss**.

We gain weight only in one place. That is inside our heads.

But it shows on our entire body.

99.99% of content on the subject of weight loss is geared towards the physicality of weight loss. It's convenient to paste a picture of a hot model on a magazine cover and attach some catchy slogan to grab your attention. I have mentioned a few of those to you. Social media preys on our fears. I have dared to use my example in this entire conversation because I have been a victim to that guile and disguise. Most of us lose our precious resources in our pursuit of good health and bodies. But more than resources we lose self-respect. We live with a feeling of self-doubt because we failed to lose weight. Something which sounds so smooth and straight forward is the leading cause of disease and misery all over the world.

I have seen relationships fail due to loss of physical attraction between 2 individuals, marriages break down, society looks down upon you if you don't fit into a stereotype set by the society, you might be superseded due to your looks, it becomes a challenge to find the right partner if you are overweight. It seems that our entire society revolves around a stereotype about how you should look. If this is so important for the way, our society operates then why don't governments put a stop to everything which leads to obesity?

All I discovered in my journey was that my health and my life were my responsibility. Multinationals will keep selling junk food, and people will keep falling sick. In my later years, as a lifestyle coach, most of the weight gain cases were actually cases with psychological issues. I have met scores of people who consume performance-enhancing products like shakes and pills while they chase an elusive body image. I know a few who have gone under the knife to lose weight. It should just make us stop and ask, "all this. For what? "

Just as in my case, one has to have the right purpose of achieving any goal. My intention was plain and straight forward. My physical health was in the hazardous territory. If I hadn't taken corrective steps to fix my health, my life was in a severe threat. If not death then for sure highly compromised and diseased. That was not an outcome acceptable to me, so I achieved what I set out for. I was fortunate to have found the right help at the right time. But everyone is not that fortunate. People don't have the resources to get the type of support I afforded to myself. On top of that, we have social media ready to pounce on our vulnerabilities and fears.

I go through a lot of content on weight loss and well-being on a daily basis. Most of it is geared to try to sell you some expensive product or enrol you in a program. It's a well-oiled machine. I have seen people paying a fortune to get hold of hunger-suppressing pills. I have seen young and fittest of people falling dead for no reason, I have seen people bulking up in a matter of weeks. They are not bothered by the consequences of taking steroids and performance-enhancing substances on their longterm health. All revolving around certain stereotypes and fears. In this entire personal journey, not once did I consume anything which came even remotely close to what I have just mentioned. Once I gained a fair understanding of the functioning of my body, I went about the task of fixing it.

I have maintained the same weight for the last 8 years now (it swings between 87 kgs and 90 kgs).

Was it a challenge in doing so?

Were there dangers of falling back into the same abyss?

Am I doing anything special to maintain that level of health?

Am I still following that manic workout regime?

These are the type of questions posed to me when I conduct my workshops and training. I am sure the same questions are already doing the rounds in your brain. The answers to these very questions are in the remaining part of our conversation. What you have with you till now is a physical part of any transformation. It's time for the psychology of weight loss now. People think of weight loss as a physical event only. They are so wrong.

You just don't appear fat. **You feel fat in your thoughts**. And anyone who is not fat simply can't understand that. It's one thing to lecture and write about weight loss. If you have not felt it in your head, then all your knowledge about weight loss is like a body without a soul. There are hardly any trainers who have experienced being fat. And that's the biggest reason why their clients either don't lose weight or regain the lost weight as soon as they are by themselves. I have not met Seb for 7 years now. I am still maintaining the weight we achieved as a team.

Let's talk about those 7 years now and how you can fix your weight problem permanently. I did not need a Seb after those 4 months. I am indebted to him for what he gave me. But post that it was all about me.

"Imagine your mind like a garden, and your thoughts are the seeds. You get to choose what seeds you plant in it. You can plant seeds of positivity, love and abundance. Or you can plant seeds of negativity, fear and lack. You can also spend time trying to take care of everyone else's garden. Or you can work on making yours beautiful and attract other beautiful people to your garden"

JAKE WOODARD

CHAPTER FIVE

OH MY GOD, THE WEIGHT IS COMING BACK

So here I was. Sort of a brand new person. A poster boy of sorts. I was full of life and energy after what I had achieved. After all, losing 36 kgs was no mean achievement. My daily routine was firmly anchored around fitness. I was not a fitness freak, but I was extremely regular and disciplined with my routine and diet. Though post my weight-loss mission, I did offer myself the luxury of treating myself occasionally with a treat here and there. But nothing catastrophic. I had understood the calorie thing completely. I knew what my BMR was. So I knew how much and what I could consume.

Another thing I did was to open a health account in the **CALORIE BANK**.

Now you must be wondering what this CALORIE BANK is?

This is a concept I developed for myself based upon my research about the calories in food items.

Now how does this work?

Simple. Just like a bank.

Say you have a savings account in any bank. This account will hold the money you deposit into the account. Every time you need some money, you will go to the ATM or the bank branch and withdraw the sum you need. If there is sufficient money in your account, then you will get what you have asked for.

Suppose you have $1000 in your account and there is a requirement of some cash. So you go to the ATM. If this requirement is up to $1000, then there is no issue. But if your need is of $1001. We have a problem even if its $1 over what you have in your saving, your request will not be serviced.

I know the quick question bubbling inside your head.

What if I have an overdraft facility? Well, this bank takes care of that as well. Because you are the owner of this bank, we trust that you will not let your bank collapse with jumbo loans.

So what does all this mean?

This was for such situations where you tend to go a bit overboard. It could be an invite to a friends place or an office gathering. There are so many situations we encounter to flounder. But don't worry. This bank keeps you in check.

Most of the social engagements are planned. You will

know beforehand when you have been invited. Let's say you have been asked for dinner on the weekend, which is three days away. You very well know that you will end up eating extra calories and empty calories.

I followed a straightforward rule.

1 BLANK CALORIE = 3 EXTRA CALORIES.

Don't try to google for this calculator. This was my personal bank, and it has worked well since the last seven years and thousands of success stories around the same concept.

I used to do something more. I used to start banking calories in my CALORIE BANK, at least two days in advance of the party.

So let's take a real-time situation.

Its a Thursday and I have received an invite for Saturday evening.

So I have two and a half days before the party—Thursday, Friday and half of Saturday.

I would start banking calories from Thursday. Not much. Just 200 calories types. I would proactively reduce my calorie intake.

Calories in bank in 2.5 days

200 X 2.5 = 500 calories.

Now come Saturday evening, and I end up consuming:

500 extra calories (normal ones)

300 blank calories (the ones with alcohol and deserts)

The total extra calories consumed:

500 + (3x 300) = 1400 extra calories.

I had 500 calories in my bank. So excess withdrawn:

1400-500 = 900 calories.

I had a rule with myself that I am allowed two days to pay back the excess withdrawn. Following this rule, I would create a negative calorie intake of 900 calories over the next two days. All this meant was a reduced diet and an intense workout.

My friend trust me on this. This single rule has helped me maintain my weight for seven years. I lead a very happening social life. There is a lot of travel involved in my work due to my business of wellness. I meet friends, family and clients regularly. My calorie bank has stood the test of time. I have taught this concept to thousands of people over the last few years. Anyone who has followed this has not gained weight after dropping it. But it was a rule which I made for myself, and it was my responsibility to adhere to it. Of course, there are many such tools I developed to maintain a healthy lifestyle. I will discuss shortly.

But something else started happening with me however. I was maintaining a very healthy lifestyle for the next few months but my mind started wandering again. Somewhere deep down, my healing was not complete. Canberra was where all my memories with my family were. Every now and then they would ambush me. There used to be weak moments. Post my personal training stint with Seb; I continued with my gym routine. But within a few months, I had started missing some sessions. In the beginning, I thought that I was just complacent and nothing more. Every now and then I would consume some junk food. I would work on the calorie bank concept. But soon I started missing my calorie deposit limit of 2 days. I would get wine and consume it beyond the limits I had set for myself. As a result of all this, I gained about 6 kgs in 6 months. It was a steady rise of about a kilo per month. The worst part of this was that despite knowing the complete process, I was not able to pull back this weight gain. The first sign of alarm was my waist. Remember how it had become 34". It increased to 36". Not much but I knew something was wrong.

Does this sound familiar? The feeling?

I had all the tools with me now. Let's recap them:

Experience to loose weight first hand.

The knowledge behind weight loss.

Tools to manage situations.

Diet plans to manage weight.

THEN WHY WAS I RE-GAINING WEIGHT?

Did this mean I would need professional help again to

reign in this bulge?

"So I would need to keep apportioning resources all my life to maintain a good weight", I would say to myself.

That was not an option with me because it was not financially sustainable. Then why is this happening again with me? I would keep pondering over this question.

One good thing during this short phase was that I did not miss the telltale signs of me slipping back into a sort of toxicity. I knew I had to hit the core of this. I did not panic this time. I was extremely observant (metacognitive) of my thoughts. I started noticing the patterns of my mood swings. I observed that whenever I saw a place which I had visited with my family, I would feel a bit low. That profound feeling would stay with me for a short time. But it was long enough to cause some damage. Like, I missed my gym sessions on a few occasion. And it was invariably after such an event. There were many notations on similar lines. So I knew that my emotional hurt had not healed. It was only bandaged. My physicality had been fixed but not my emotional health. It was still some distance from being healed.

At work, front things were good. I had managed to make a very small saving for myself. I was trying to get a bigger role for myself in my organisation. But that was not happening. It was largely due to the reason of Canberra being a smaller city than say Sydney or Melbourne.

What to do now?

I started toying with a thought of moving out from Canberra to Sydney or Melbourne. It was just a thought at that stage. I knew what it meant to move out of Canberra. Let me list it out for you:

Moving to a place where you didn't know a soul.

Much bigger cities. So increased expenses.

The expense to make an interstate move.

I was moving away from my children.

These were serious points to consider. The organisation I was working at that time did not promote interstate transfers. So that was not an option either.

I worked out a plan. It was a very long shot. But I remembered the incident at the car agency. I didn't have any hope of saving my car, but things happened.

I spoke to myself.

 "You have a very good experience as a manager. Your KPI's are extremely good. You have very sound references. There is no harm in trying".

Kindly observe the self-talk here. How it was all toxic and devoid of any optimism earlier, it was now all about possibilities and optimism. So I decided to apply for jobs in both Sydney and Melbourne. This kept me busy for the next couple of weeks. I started getting calls for job interviews from both Sydney and Melbourne. The initial conversations would all go well and move to the next level. It is here where I hit a roadblock. My resume was solid, and it was a perfect fit for the job descriptions of the positions I had applied for, except for one thing. I was not living in those cities, and usually, people don't move interstate without a preeminent reason. Almost all leads dried out except for a couple. Even from those leads, there was no further communication. They were as good as dried up.

So was this the end of my audacious plan?

This time I was not giving up so easily. I had climbed an almost impossible mountain just a few months back. So I backed myself. I knew the odds of getting an appropriate job in these megacities were very slim while I was in Canberra. The odds would become really good if I applied for these jobs if I was living in these cities. It was back to the drawing board.

Out came my diary. I started calculating the expenses of living in these cities. I would check online about rents and leases. Food was more or less the same. Then I looked at my savings. I matched the two. I had enough to sustain myself without a job, for about three months. Not a lot but still something to ponder on. I slept on this for a few days. Honestly, I felt scared to jump into this. But I had made up my mind to jump. I decided to put in my papers and move to Melbourne. There was shock at my workplace. My boss was seriously concerned about my well being. He tried to talk me out of this, but I had decided. There was a notice period in my contract, so it was still sometime before I finally left Canberra.

As the date of my notice period came close, the reality started sinking in. I had not lived at any other place other than Canberra ever since I had migrated to Australia.

Now let me narrate the funny part in this. You must be thinking why Melbourne and not Sydney.

Remember how I had received many interview calls in the initial stage. And gradually all leads had dried up except for a couple. There was one lead from Melbourne and two from Sydney which were technically still open. So simple logic says that I should have gone to Sydney as there were two leads from there. In my mind, these leads had also dried up because there was no communication from any of these. But still, why Melbourne? It was certainly not a toss of the coin here. You know I was born in India. And cricket is vast in India and Australia. As a child, I always had this fascination for the boxing day test match at the MCG. The Melbourne cricket ground. So I said to myself, "Vineet lets go to Melbourne". And it was Melbourne.

As my departure date approached, there was this mixed feeling of sadness, excitement and suspense. I had started packing my belongings in boxes. One particular day, as I sat on the floor, there was everything material I owned packed in a few boxes. My entire collection boxed up. It was a very profound moment. I did not have a lot of things. But whatever I had, was bought with a lot of love. All the boxes were given to the packers and movers for delivery to an address in Melbourne. I had rented a small place after a little research. The criteria were safety and the ease of accessibility to the city centre. I had no idea about how this megacity was designed. All I knew was that it was voted as the worlds most liveable city, and there was MCG.

Finally, the day came for my journey to Melbourne. I decided to drive down to Melbourne. It was a 12-hour drive with a few stoppages for rest. This was my first drive of that distance and duration. I had a GPS with me. So I put the designated address in it. I worked out that a safe time to start my journey would be a very early morning start. I wanted to reach my destination early evening. I picked up a route crisscrossing the south coast. This route was lined with a few significant towns. I thought, why not drive through them. It will just give me some visual treats. So I started at 4 am. Made a pit stop just on Canberra borders to top up fuel, for one last time, for my car and some eats for myself. The feeling was something which took me a couple of years to process. It was a feeling of driving my purpose. Something inside me was reassuring me—the same small feeble voice. I drove on and hit the highway and hit the cruise control.

110 km an hour.

The Australian roads are the best when it comes to quality. I have been fortunate for having an opportunity to visit many countries in Europe, Asia and America. The roads in Australia are right amongst the top. With my favourite music in the background, I was cutting my chords with some very uncomfortable memories. With one audacious act of stepping out of my comfort zone, I could feel those memories losing their power of causing damage to me. I was in an excellent mood. Coffee. Music. Beautiful visuals. Hope. And a sandwich of coarse. I was following the verbal instructions from the GPS and just flying. It felt as if the wheels of my car were not in contact with the metal road. It was a lovely liberated feeling.

I reached a town called Bega. It must have been about 10 am. My mobile rang. Who would call me now? I just thought. I was a bit irritated as the call broke the dream sequence I was in. You know, songs, coffee, suspense, plans type of dream sequence. I just glanced at my phone and couldn't recognise the number. It was not a stored number. I just slowed down and pulled up on the dirt track on the side of the highway. I took the call with the customary greeting. The voice on the other side was that of a girl, and she said," Vineet, our HR head would like to have a conversation with you regarding the role you had applied with us. Your application has moved to the final stage. Is this a good time to talk ?". It was a call from the company in Melbourne where I had applied for.

I simply couldn't believe what I had just heard. I responded in the affirmative, and the call was transferred to the HR head. The conversation continued for about 45 minutes. For the entire duration of this conversation, I had not mentioned that I was sitting in my car, on a highway, my belongings packed for Melbourne and myself a few hours from the city. We reached the final stages of this conversation, and I was asked a very pointed question. It was about my availability. The lady was pleasantly taken aback when I informed that I was on my way to Melbourne and would be available to join at the shortest notice. Greetings were exchanged again, and the conversation ended. I let out a big gasp of air from my mouth.

Now, this was not ordinary by any chance. At that particular moment, I was plain happy. I couldn't process the event any more than that. But was it just a series of coincidences or was it something else.

I knew that the level for which I had applied, the HR head calls only if they have shortlisted you for the role. And I was sure about another thing, that if they have called me up then probably I am the only candidate left who satisfies the role description. Remember, I was not in Melbourne when I had applied. And I must have not been the first choice just due to that reason. Anyways, now I was on a different gear altogether. Wow. I was on the cusp of finding a brand new job in a brand new city. How good was that? The remainder of the drive became even more pleasurable. The distance remained the same, but the time got shorter. Sometime before the evening, I hit the highway into Melbourne.

I still remember my first visions of this megacity. It's different, and I had not experienced anything of the sorts before. Six lane highways. Massive logistic trucks. Tall skyscrapers. I was enjoying this. In the midst of all this, I reached the place I had rented. I had made a call to the contact person once I had entered Melbourne. So he was there to hand me the keys and sign a few documents. Once settled in my new place, the next few days went like a breeze. I was exploring the suburb for the shopping areas and just generally getting a feel of this beautiful city. Of course, there was not a soul I could call as I knew no one.

"I went looking for Him And lost myself; The drop merged with the sea - Who can find it now ?"
SAINT KABIR.

It must have been a week later that I received a call from the place I had applied for. This time I could recognise the number as I had fed it in my contact list. It was the same voice with whom I had the initial conversation on the highway. I was informed that my application had moved to the final stage. That stage is when they do the police and reference checks. I knew I had got the job. It would be a move up the ladder in terms of the role. The take-home salary would be higher than my previous job. My bold step seemed to have worked.

It was not long that I received the call which I had been waiting for. It was an in-person meeting with the regional head for the final salary negotiations. All of that had happened in quick succession, and within a fortnight of my reaching Melbourne, I had my professional life firmly anchored with an outstanding job.

I loved the role. I loved the city. The routine was no different from the one I was following in Canberra. The only small challenge was the long distance between my workplace and home. It would take me in excess of two and a half hours driving to work and back. This was a big chunk of my time taken away. So as I priority, I relocated to someplace closer to work. This took about three months to achieve. The period we are conversing about now is early 2014. A lot of water had flown under the bridge since 2010 till now.

My move to this new place really opened up a lot of hours for me. My workout regime was back in place. There would be no more ambushes by well-known sites like the one in Canberra. So emotionally, I was way better. I started to get a handle on my weight again. It was back to the levels which I had achieved with Seb.

Something else commenced in this period. Something very innocuous and innocent.

I had started connecting with old friends through social media. And it was a wonderful experience. It really killed my isolation and that isolation was replaced by chats with friends, discussions about my weight loss and many pleasant topics. Being in Australia gave me a 5 hour 30 minutes heads up due to the time zone difference between the two countries. This was a very convenient difference. I would return from my gym workout in the evening and then connect with a few friends late in the evening Melbourne time. It would still be noon time in India. There would be laughter, jokes, stories and fun in these interactions. My friends would encourage me to visit India for a holiday. I had not met any one of those childhood friends since close to 30 years. The boys had turned into middle-aged men. But the friendships remained boyish. Those friendships were untouched by the journey of life.

The bodies had signs of individual struggles and tribulations. But the bonds were still young, innocent and fresh. It really felt good every time I would connect with some friend. Someone would always be available for a chat every evening. They were all amazed at my transformation. I used to share my pictures and routines with them. Some would ask for help and guidance to get their health on track. I would share everything I had learnt in this time. After all, these were childhood friends. In fact, I used to look forward to these interactions with them in the evening. I would also text them during my breaks at work and follow up. It was the same routine which Seb followed with me. Remember how he used to text me during the day and just let me know that big brother is watching. The only difference here was that I would incessantly text my poor friends. I could take those liberties as these were buddies. There was no professional wall of formality to reckon with. There was a sense of pleasure while doing this. It also had connotations of responsibility to help them regain their health. Many would start some kind of a routine, but then they would fall back to their same old habits—some within a few hours and Some within a few days. But there were a very few, two or three, who persisted much longer than that. They started following my suggestions, and we could see fantastic results.

To start with, they were not facing the sort of a challenge which I did. So it was relatively more straightforward for us to get some results in a short time. This was incredibly inspiring and provided me with a lot of satisfaction.

An improvement in the health of someone else was providing me with self-satisfaction. What I did not register was that this was the beginning of a new chapter in my life. Absolutely unaware but I was taking baby steps towards coaching. For me, it was just a satisfying task which I used to look forward to. But remember that I was dealing with childhood friends. Some of these relationships went back for more than 4 decades. There was no room for any formality or commercial arrangement in this.

I went on doing this for a couple of weeks when one of my friends asked me something which I had neither factored nor thought about. He asked if I would help a person who was a very good friend of his, to lose weight.

This was a situation of helping someone whom I didn't know personally. I did not find anything wrong in that until my friend put in another caveat to this. He said," **you should charge him something**". Now, this was something I had not dealt with ever. I had always hired people or paid consultancies but never had I charged a consultancy from anyone. I was a mid-level manager working in a multinational. My favourite date on the calendar used to be the 1st Friday of every month. As that was pay day for me. I had not experienced receiving money in any other way. I tried to wriggle out of the situation by giving many reasons, but my friend was insistent on the money part.

Somewhere I was getting convinced that if there is a **service rendered, then there should be a charge associated** with that service. With a promise that I would think about the proposal, we brought an end to that conversation.

A COACH IS BORN BY CHANCE

We reconnected, and I proposed a very benign figure to render my coaching services to this person whom I had never met or spoken. I did not know how he looked like. All I knew was that he was friends with my friend, had some weight issues and was very keen to be helped by me. This keenness was fired by the results he saw on my friend and of course the upselling by my friend.

Mobile numbers were exchanged courtesy the shared link. A convenient time was set up for a voice talk. This would be the very first time I would be speaking to someone as a trainer. This was unknown territory for me—unchartered waters. I did feel the presence of some sort of pressure in my thoughts. I found it to be funny and scary. Nevertheless, we spoke, and the entire conversation was around the issues the person was facing. Unknowingly I was incorporating all my learnings with Seb by default. I took all the details painstakingly. A separate note was created on my desktop. I asked all those questions which used to be inside me when I was going through the same issues. We discussed the charges which were minuscule as compared to what I had paid or even as compared to what was being charged in India. Making money was not intent in this. The presence of a fee was to make this look a serious affair. And it did that job pretty effectively. I had a dormant savings account in India, and I used this account to get a transfer from my first client. A tiny but such an important event. This was the milestone which I look back upon with a great sense of pride and benevolence. An act where the intent was solely rooted in an innocent act of helping someone to regain health, became the starting point for the most significant change in my life. I did not see it like that when it happened. But today, years after it unfolded, when I process the chain of events leading to that point, it is amply clear to me how my actions were deciding my future. I have no doubt over that.

I made a detailed routine for my first client regarding his diet and daily routine.

Here's the funny part. Now that I had someone to train professionally, it became like a life mission of sorts. And please keep in mind that I had a time zone lead of 5.5 hours over this gentleman and all of this was happening remotely over text messaging, emails and video calling. I used this with aplomb and was all over my client. He had not experienced anything like this before. I would expect him to send me texts on everything I had asked him to do.

For me it was simple,

You eat something. Send a picture of what you ate.

You go for a walk. Send the picture of the pedometer.

You don't eat anything on time. You will get a text from me.

Everything around the routine had to be recorded in texts. On returning home, I would speak to him and encourage him. We struck an excellent working relationship.

Results were slow, as expected, but they were there. I could predict with a fair accuracy about those results. I would share the knowledge I had gained in my journey, and this really helped us to find common ground.

Within the next 3 weeks, my client had lost 6 kgs of weight, and it showed. People around him starting noticing and complimenting on his success. Both of us shared this sense of joy and achievement.

For me, it was the first taste of success of a methodology of remote training.

For my client, it was the taste of success of winning a battle which he had lost a few time previously.

This routine continued for three months, and my first client ended up shedding 15 kgs in that time. It was a resounding success. Both of us gained tremendously. Confidence was sky-high. My client became a walking and talking brochure of my services by default. His transformation was so stark and distinct that people around him started enquiring about how he achieved such results. By the end of 3 months, I had another three clients whom I was training remotely from Melbourne. All of these clients were in Delhi.

My evenings and weekends changed forever. Being at a senior level in my organisation, there was a lot of responsibility for my role. So I had to make use of my evenings in the most productive fashion. My previous interactions with friends had now become professional exchanges with remote clients. There was this responsibility and drive to get results. My weekends were the most hectic. I was making the most effective use of the time zones. I would finish my weekly grocery shopping and my own workout in the morning time. By midday, I would be ready for my clients in India. I was incessant in my followups and suggestions. There was no scope of a slip-up. My own research into health also picked up pace and direction. I was really enjoying this experience.

BUT IT WAS STILL A HOBBY TYPE OF ACTIVITY. I HAD NOT EVEN REMOTELY THOUGHT ABOUT MAKING THIS A CAREER.

I was not chasing any clients. Nor was I concerned about what I was being paid. A small amount was getting collected, and I always thought that this would help me in a small way whenever I decide to go on holiday to India. Nothing more at that point.

But what started as friendly advice to my friends had by now turned into a piece of structured professional advice to clients. By the end of 2014, I had trained about 20 clients in India. The results were 100%. I had followed the same strategy with all of them. But each one had a totally personalised program. **It was not a cut-copy-paste approach**. Every fresh client was the result of the outcome of the previous client. It was all happening by word of mouth publicity. At an average, I was taking on 5 to 8 fresh people on board each month. It was becoming serious work by the end of 2014. I had to politely refuse some people as my evenings and weekends were getting jam-packed with clients, and there was a limit as to how many people I could communicate with within those hours. The small amounts were all adding up in my account in India.

I distinctly remember that it was late December 2014 and it was a particularly tiring Christmas season for us. Christmas is a crucial period for anyone who is in retail in Australia. And we had a really good season. Our bonuses are made or broken at this time.

I had a few days to relax post that and I drove down to the GREAT OCEAN ROAD near Melbourne. I just wanted to relax and unwind. I was in a particularly useful frame of mind: a well-executed season and the satisfaction of training so many people. I was lapping up the visual treats of this great city. My move to Melbourne had paid off. My health was in control, and my career was in much better shape.

A thought just brushed my consciousness. It was about the possibility of taking up wellness training more seriously and augmenting it as a second job. It was a thought which made all sense as I had tasted some success during the last few months. It felt delicious and reassuring. I kept toying with this thought on my way back from the drive. It is a 2-hour drive, and I really did not notice how that time elapsed. I was so engrossed and engaged with that thought. I thought of bouncing this idea with a few close friends in Australia and India. **We all look for validation for our beliefs**. I was no different. I received a lot of encouragement from everyone I spoke. But these were my well-wishers.

Invariably all of them asked one pointed question. It was about my current job and my financial security in the context of quitting this well-paying job and jumping onto something which was more of a hobby. I found merit in those questions. But I could not miss the telltale signs of the satisfaction I derived while training people. Though it was all done remotely, the results and financial gains were all too distinct to be ignored or overlooked. So I did what I always did.....

GET THE NUMBERS RIGHT. PLAN PLAN AND PLAN.

I took a conscious decision that I would not make any decision in haste. An opportunity had presented itself to me inadvertently, and I was in no mood to ignore it or rush into it.

"Creating meaning involves bringing order to the contents of the mind by integrating one's actions into a unified flow"
MIHALY CSIKSZENTMIHALYI.

My financial state was much better than what it used to be while I was in Canberra. However, better is a comparative word. It certainly looked better when compared to what it was. Still nothing flush or extravagant. Just comfortable. So I put a straightforward plan in place.

I was now chasing a feeling of purpose. And I wanted this feeling to replace my current state of activities, income, career and direction of my life. That's a lot of changes to reckon with. I listed a few things in my notes book.

1. **Was I really looking at something real, or was I creating a scenario with my imagination?**
2. **What would it take to really make this something real and long term?**
3. **What sort of training do I require to do justice for a new career?**
4. **What was the market size for a newbie like myself?**
5. **Would I still get the same enjoyment if I took this as a full-time career option?**
6. **How would the numbers match up when it comes to taking care of my expenses.**
7. **Do I just want to be another trainer, or was I chasing something different?**
8. **Do I really want to do this?**

There were so many questions to grapple with, and they didn't have simple, straightforward answers. I required a plan. And I got down to do the same. I had to give it an earnest thought if I wanted to turn this into a profession from just a hobby. I welcomed the new year with all these thoughts and questions and possibilities.

DO YOU REALISE THAT WE HAVE TRAVELLED FROM 2010 TO 2015.

Five years encapsulated over a few hours.

What used to be a challenge to survive in 2010 had now transformed into an opportunity.

Those moments of total despair had been replaced by moments of excitement.

The self-talk had changed from **survival to fulfilment.**

I put in place a plan to address all the questions which would help me to make an informed decision regarding my future. Its summarised here for us:

1. I would keep giving 100% to my current job. No compromise with that because that would put a question mark on my **integrity**.

2. I would raise my charges to a realistic level so that I can come to a lifelike picture with my hobby. Till now, my charges were highly discounted as compared to the market rates on anything similar going around.

3. I would give more **structure** to the training modules.

4. I will rejoin professional training to **upgrade** my knowledge.

5. I will do intensive **research** on the subject of wellness.

6. I will **network** to create **resources** which were paramount for **the success** of a business.

7. I will **simulate** scenarios so that my **planning** has most things factored in.

If you take notice, I was working on specific concepts, which are a bedrock of any successful business model. The first step I took was to create a buffer zone between my existing clients and any new signups. There used to be constant requests for taking on fresh people. But I kept refusing politely. I then worked out a realistic and sustainable fee for my services. It was much higher than what I was charging till that time. But it was still lower than the prevailing market rates. **This one single step would decide if this would remain as a hobby or if it was destined**

for something much more significant and formidable.

On receiving the next request for training, I quoted the new figure. There was absolutely no trace of anxiety within me on the outcome. After all, I was finding an answer to an earnest question of my life. It's better to face reality rather than being in a dream sequence.

I signed up a fresh client within a few days. However, the number of new clients dwindled to 2 or 3 for the first two months. But this was at a very realistic rate. To my satisfaction, the number of signups was back to the figures of 6 to 8 within the next few months. This one step **morphed my hobby into a serious career option**. By the month of April 2015, I was dealing with the same number of clients as before. I was working on all the points I had listed out for myself.

THERE WAS A PURPOSE IN MY ROUTINE NOW.

I was now executing a plan which was well thought out and structured. There was nothing random in this. One step was to lead to the next. I had kept a milestone in this plan. This is interesting now.

I had accrued an annual leave of 4 weeks in my leave account by now. For the uninitiated, this is a paid leave entitlement with every employee of the organisation. I sent in a request of 2 weeks of annual leave in the month of August 2015. This was approved by my bosses. Now came a very critical step in my entire journey. I wanted to travel to India in these two weeks. The foremost reason was to conduct a live seminar on wellness in India and come face to face with prospective clients. The secondary purpose was to meet my friends after a gap of more than three decades. I had a comfortable saving to finance this trip. I again took help from my friends and booked a top-rated facility in Delhi for my first ever seminar. I circulated my itinerary with all my current and past clients to invite prospective clients for this health talk. I was to travel in the 3rd week of august, and the date for my first seminar was **23rd of August 2015, Delhi.**

I carefully created a PowerPoint presentation for the purpose. I designed the signage for the show. I created the invites. All of this was happening while I was in Melbourne.

I travelled to India in mid of August. Meeting my family and friends was an emotional moment. I had locked everyone out of my life at one point in my life. And now I was reconnecting with everyone. There were tears, and there were bear hugs. A part of me healed instantly. I realised the importance of these connects and the gross mistake I had committed by moving away from them. It was also time to celebrate this reunion, and I did celebrate that. I remember that there was just about a week in between my landing and the seminar. The groundwork done over the past few weeks had paid off. There was very little left in terms of preparation for the seminar.

I had never conducted a seminar prior to this. I had been a part of many corporate pieces of training but never a solo act. So this was a bit unnerving for me. I was getting some sleepless nights. It was not because of the content. **IT WAS ABOUT ME**.

Will I be able to make an excellent presentation?

Will I be able to connect with people?

Will I be able to convince people that remote training works?

I had all such questions running amok in my thoughts. I checked and then double-checked all the preparations. I ran the presentation in my mind over and over again.

I WAS IN A ZONE.

A day prior to the seminar date, I lost all my anxiety and fear. I simply went about socialising with friends and family. On the morning of 23rd, I was ready to deliver the seminar by 8 am the scheduled timing was 10 am.

IT WAS SHOWTIME.

I did not have a PR company to run this for me. Nor did I have a team to check or do anything. But I had some friends who stood as rocks with me in this. There were 5 of them. They divided the work of welcoming the guests to the venue and getting them seated. They put up the signages in a melody like a sequence. They were giving instructions to the hospitality staff. I was also there. I would meet numerous clients for the very first time. It was a unique experience. Even now it's bringing a smile. Some were very formal. A few very emotional. A few outright excited. The energy at the venue was very high. There were laughs and smiles all around. It almost descended into a party zone. Exactly at 9.50 am, I heard my voice for the very first time on a sound system. I requested everyone to take their seat. I have delivered in excess of 300 talks since that date. But that feeling remains unmatched. **The talk commenced**. It had moments of fun. It had a few disciplining moments. The PowerPoint presentation went through seamlessly. I connected with the entire audience of about 120 people. There were small activities to bring home certain aspects of wellness. I conducted on the spot quizzes. Something that was planned as a 3-hour session, refreshment break included, stretched to 4 hours. Time simply accelerated. Each person in that hall could feel the energy. My maiden attempt to organise a show had been a resounding success. By the time I was left with just those five friends of mine, it was close to 4 pm in the evening.

By the time I woke up the next morning, **I had been approached by 35 participants for personalised wellness programs.** This was way beyond anything I had planned for. If someone asked me at that time," did I ever imagine this ?".

The answer was an emphatic "no".

There was a sense of accomplishment. But there was this sense of responsibility which came with such a response. I very well understood what it meant.

I had also planned for a short holiday to Goa, a vibrant tourist place on the western coast of India. This was my first true holiday in 15 years. Lots of firsts. Little did I know that those few days spent on the beautiful beaches of Goa would translate into something else, a few months down the line.

The remaining days in India were spent interacting with this fresh batch of clients. A new class of 35 people. Never before had I interacted with such a large number of clients at one time. It required a lot of planning and the most important was of time management. If I say that I got busy after this, it would be an understatement. I was super busy. On my return to Melbourne, I had to reschedule my entire day. With my primary job still being a non-negotiable, I had to apportion my time before and after work. I was genuinely working two jobs now. I was trying to do justice to both of them. Most of the days, I would work late into the nite as I had to fit in this clutch of signups. I was totally consumed by work. I had the same 24 hours as before. But I had to squeeze more out of these hours. So I had to continually tweak the rules of engagement. I was working with close to 50 individual programs. The financial gains were extremely good. I was making really good money along with my regular job. Sometime in November, the pressure of the new Christmas season descended upon me. I had to reckon with the extra effort required for the season and my fledgling business. I used to feel the physical crunch of working close to 20 hours a day. There was no time for my own workouts or training. I was reaching a breaking point in terms of the physicality involved. But I did not give in. The pressure resulted in better structure and scheduling of my engagements.

There was this realisation that my regular job required more effort from my side. It was after all a job. And my business required much less effort as I used to **enjoy doing it**. Even after a full day worth of work with my primary job, I used to look forward to the evening and the sense of satisfaction I derived out of it. The year was on wheels. I had reached Christmas 2015 from 2014. The year 2015 was a defining one for me professionally. **It had opened up an avenue which was purpose-driven.**

It seemed I had stumbled upon my **purpose in life.**

But first things first. I had to get through the season. My integrity towards my job was a non-negotiable. I always remembered what this job gave me and the responsibility I was holding. So I purposely toned down the consultancy to a level which I could manage without compromising on my delivery on both fronts. I put on hold any new sign up for the entire month of December. This really helped. I could get through the seasonal sale period and also give the best possible guidance to all my clients. I was getting an excellent handle on the concept of time management now. I would remember these lessons for the new phase of my life, which I was about to enter.

My emotional state was of accomplishment and satisfaction. There was no place of any self-defeating talks or any hurt from the past. I was making peace with my past. I could not find a reason why things were happening the way they were. And neither could I find a reason to the way things had happened in the not so distant past. We always think that we are in control of what we are doing.

What I mean is that we think that we are consciously doing things. **This is a myth which got shattered** later in my life and gave me a brand new perspective about concepts such as fate and destiny. More on that shortly.

Another season came and went away smoothly.

Once again, I was driving on the Great Ocean Road.

This time I was to make an important decision in my life. I knew that I could not do these two jobs simultaneously. I had been fortunate that both were getting executed well. But I knew that it was not possible for me to physically accomplish both things. What was only a hobby precisely a year ago, was now running parallel to the main job—both in terms of the financial returns and the time consumed.

But it was winning in one aspect. **IT WAS WAY MORE SATISFYING**.

I was now veering around the notion of getting involved full-time in this newfound passion. But I talked myself to be more patient. The start of 2016 was electric in terms of the number of signups happening. It was a steady stream, and I started extrapolating the time devoted to this passion and the results obtained. It was crystal clear to me that if I gave it all of my time, then the results would be even more fantastic. There was no doubt about that. I kept up my own training side by side. I was getting equipped with knowledge and tools which could help people. Planning was vital in this entire journey. Regardless of the resources at your disposal, if you have a good plan, then your odds of success rise manifolds.

A good plan backed by a passion for following through is difficult to beat.

So what did I do?

What I always do. Back to the drawing board.

This time it was a bit different though. It was not about survival.

There was no experimentation. I had done all of that.

I knew that there was a need for trainers.

I had lots of self-confidence.

I knew my methodology was unique, and it was passion-driven.

I required capital, and I didn't have lots of it.

With these pointers, I started doing a **mental rehearsal** of the entire process. I was not overconfident at any given moment. I was cognizant of the fact that I was in my late forties and the market was flooded with way younger and fitter trainers. What were the odds of my success in such a scenario? I kept on pondering about this.

Was there anything special that I could learn or do to have an edge?

The issue was of scaling up the present model and give it longevity. I kept reminding myself of one crucial thing.

"Vineet, you are enjoying doing this. So go full steam into this only if you think that you will keep enjoying doing this." This was my self-talk.

I knew that I had reached a **CROSSROAD** in my life. An opportunity had presented itself to me. It was an opportunity to realise the **PURPOSE** of my life. To give my life meaning.

To find the meaning of "meaning".

I had arrived at that crossroads due to a chain of events. And I started observing the patterns of such events. They were unmissable. I was almost 50 years of age at that point.

I simply said to myself," if not now, then when".

This settled the issue. It put my mind at rest. The self-talk was not about, "should I or shouldn't I". It was more about "let's plan". I would mentally rehearse the process. Calculations were made and scratched and made again. I bounced my plan off a few people. Took valuable inputs. I surfed the net for details about the various business models doing the rounds in Australia and India. As usual, I was planning hard. I had limited resources. So I had to ensure that these resources work harder and last longer.

It had just been a couple of years into my job in Melbourne. I had made some good friends over there. I discussed this wild idea of mine with my boss. Of course, he was taken aback. But everyone supported me. That way, I am fortunate to be in a culture where innovation and risk-taking go hand in hand. People support your ideas without any biases. I will not stretch the commentary around my final few months in the organisation as the exciting part is about to begin. I put in my papers in the march of 2016.

The plan that I had made was to conduct training seminars in India and Australia and through these seminars, sign up clients for further training. I had been doing it on a smaller scale already. So now it was just about scaling it up. I had done some calculations, and I reached a conclusion that the capital I had saved up was enough to carry me through for about 15 months even if I didn't sign up a single client during that entire time period. Obviously what it meant was a frugal living and doing most of the tasks myself. There was no room for any extravagance. Plus there would be no automatic credits going into my account on the first Friday of each month.

I WAS ON MY OWN NOW.

I was starting a new career when I was just about to hit 50 in a few years.

People use words and expressions such as self-belief, courage, will power, fate, motivation, madness, passion etc. to describe what I did. I was one of them.

But we were all wrong.

The only correct word is "purpose".

If you find purpose, then all the other words and expressions are a by-product. What I was about to see in the coming time period was the enormity of this word. Everything changed after that. And the quest for the name "purpose" came from a simple question which was extremely important for the success and longevity of my business.

"WHY DO PEOPLE FIND IT DIFFICULT TO LOSE WEIGHT?"

Our next bit of conversation will be around this question and its offshoots.

Remember," weight loss was the bedrock of my business model". The entire model was based on the premise that I can help people lose weight and get healthier. I had my own story to highlight and scores of success stories which had been created in the past few months.

What if I discovered that my model was incomplete?

What if I found that there was no longevity in the processes I had designed?

What if I found that my knowledge was incomplete?

CHAPTER SIX

THE BILLION DOLLAR HEIST AROUND WEIGHT LOSS

I had inadvertently become a part of the **"billion-dollar weight-loss industry"**. I have no doubt or fear in calling this a **HEIST**.

Now, what on earth am I speaking about? Let me explain.

A toxic narrative has been created around this weight loss "DRAMA". The narrative has statements rather than solutions, hitting the core of the issue. There is certainly no debate on the fact that weight gain is an issue and we know the implications around it. But let's list out some of the statements:

You are overweight.

- It's not good for your health.
- It's not good for the public image.

- It's easy to lose weight.
- It's all due to your lifestyle choices.
- This is the latest diet being followed by celebrities. So you do it as well.
- Oh. That diet is outdated. Now follow this one. It's the latest.
- Follow this routine. You will get motivated to lose weight.
- This is the best morning routine. Weight will start dropping off you.
- This diet is the secret of the youthfulness of sages. We have solved the mystery for you.
- This diet will reverse 20 years of ageing in a few weeks.

I can carry on listing such "statements". It's important to observe what the above statements are subtly trying to do to you. Let's start listing that now :

- plainly visible facts such as extra weight and the problems it can create. SO NO ROCKET SCIENCE REQUIRED FOR THAT.
- Instilling a feeling of being inadequate by not fitting into a body type and dress size. SO CREATING A NARRATIVE AROUND BIASED SOCIAL NORMS.
- Compelling you to compare yourself with some celebrity and how to compete with that Image. SO PITTING YOU IN A COMPETITION WITHOUT YOU EVEN BEING AWARE OF IT. MAKING YOU CHASE AN IMAGE.
- Telling you about how "wrong" is everything about your life because you don't fit into a certain size. CREATING A FEELING OF SELF DOUBT

LEADING TO LOW SELF ESTEEM.

- Telling you how easy it is to achieve weight loss. SO TELLING YOU HOW INCAPABLE YOU ARE AS YOU HAVE NOT ACHIEVED IT.

- Flashing new fads doing the rounds around the world. SO TELLING YOU THAT YOU ARE NOT UP TO DATE AND WELL INFORMED IF YOU ARE NOT A PART OF THAT LATEST FAD.

- Creating suspense around the process of weight loss. SO THAT YOU CHASE SOME QUESTION WHICH ACTUALLY HAS NO RELEVANCE IN YOUR LIFE.

- Telling you how good your life will be after you lose weight. WELL, WE ALL KNOW THAT.

- Telling you that your weight gain is the root cause of all your issues. SO THAT MEANS PEOPLE WITH THE "SUPPOSEDLY CORRECT WEIGHT" HAVE NO ISSUES.

- Selling you a dream based around an image type created via media. ITS AN IMAGE. NOT REALITY.

The reason I am listing these out is that we started this conversation around my journey of weight loss. And how things unfolded in my life. And now here I was, starting a brand new business based **EXACTLY UPON THE ABOVE MENTIONED STATEMENTS**. The obvious question you would have now is "why the hell I went into this if I knew about it in the first place?".

To answer that straightaway will not be appropriate. Let the story unfold.

I had just embarked upon a new venture, and all of my

energies were focussed in making it a success. My "primary intent" right from the beginning was to share my knowledge to help people regain their healths. If that endeavour translated into a career, then I found it absolutely legitimate. The word to take notice is "intent ".

As mentioned earlier," **I HAD BECOME A PART OF THE BILLION-DOLLAR HEIST NOW"**, though it was not intended to be like that. We have 2 questions to address here. First, why I got into this if I knew that it was a con job. Second, why people find it difficult to lose weight.

Before we proceed, I need to give you a peek into my life after I had taken the plunge into this venture.

Being born and brought up in Delhi, it should have been a foregone conclusion that my operating base, in India, would be Delhi. All my friendships and connects were Delhi based. Most of my past and current clients were Delhi based.

Remember the first seminar in August 2015? And how I had taken a small holiday to Goa after the success of that seminar. I had spent probably all of 4 days in Goa in that mini vacation. Those 4 days were enough for me to take this decision of making Goa as my operating base.

I was swept away by the idyllic beauty of the place. The raw innocence of the local population. The fresh air of the wild coconut trees. The picture-perfect beaches and the shacks serving food on those beaches. A blend of international and domestic travellers. Fantastic colonial-type cafes and eateries. I was totally sold to this. I had lived all my life in megacities such as Delhi, Nairobi, Dubai and Melbourne. This opportunity to live in an idyllic setup and continue with my work was just too good to be passed on. So it was Goa for me.

I did land in Delhi to put in place a small network to support my venture. This primarily was to service my social media account and some bit of printing work. I already had a few friends who would always crease out any logistic bumps for me. In Goa, I leased a small but furnished villa for myself in a gated community. It was very close to the beaches, and there were small markets around for my grocery needs. The place was quiet. Most of the villas were not occupied; hence there was no partying or loud music. The property was immaculately maintained, and there was more than a generous green cover. It was straight out of some picture postcard.

I would start my day at 5 a.m. with a coffee at the swimming pool within the premises. The morning chirps of the birds would greet me. I would drive down to the beaches at about 6 a.m. with my laptop and phone. They would be absolutely bereft of any human activity at that time. I had befriended the staff of a shack on that beach. So I would pull a chair and sit right on the edge of the beach where the small waves would gently roll on my bare feet. My breakfast was standard, and it would be served around 7a.m. The fresh air from the ocean would caress my face, and the cool waters of the same ocean would wash my feet. The serving of my breakfast would attract the attention of sea birds. Their loud demands for food would extract a conversation between myself and them. Some stray dogs became my companions for the morning rendezvous. And all this time my communication with my various clients would be happening.

THIS WAS MY OFFICE. SIMPLY PRICELESS

I would head back to the villa around 8 a.m. as the sun would start getting hotter. The entire day at the villa would be spent communicating with my clients. Sometimes on the stairway at the entrance of the villa and sometimes under the shade of the trees near the swimming pool. I would cook fresh meals for myself during the day. I had chosen a gym not far from where I was living. I would use the facility post-lunch. The evenings were standard. I would drive down to the beach just before the sunset and simply gaze at the majestic view of the setting sun into the shimmering ocean. The place I visited for this view was different from the one I visited in the morning. My dinner used to be at this place. It was grilled fish or chicken with fresh salad. I never carried my laptop with me in the evening. This was totally MY time. I would take long walks on the beach. Over a period of time, I befriended some regulars on the beach. It was limited to a wave of the arm or just a warm smile. I would return to the villa by 730p.m. and finish the last bits of communications with my clients.

MY ENTIRE DAY WAS A HOLIDAY, AND THE ENTIRE DAY I WOULD BE WORKING.

This was my standard routine during the week. My weekends were different. All my seminars were planned for Saturday morning. Simply because Saturday would be the day off for most people; hence they would be able to attend my seminars on their day off. I had made a circuit in which I would visit a different city each weekend. If it was Delhi one week, then it would be Kolkata the next week and Jaipur the next one and so forth. I would leave for the designated city on a Friday evening from Goa. Deliver the seminar on a Saturday morning. Spend that evening in the city and start back for Goa on a Sunday afternoon. The social media team would design campaigns accordingly, and my travel agent would have all my reservations well in advance. Sunday evening, I used to be back on the beach.

It must be appearing as a dream sequence to you. It actually was. And I lived that dream for a good 1 year. I would visit Melbourne every 4 months and conduct similar seminars. The entire plan was clicking in place. I had started thinking big in terms of scales and the opportunities available.

I was hitting very good numbers. The personal programs were getting better by the day. I could see a small army of followers on my social media handles. The capital was getting accrued. There were discussions with certain professionals for fine-tuning the strategy to take the business to the next level. Confidence was sky-high.

But something was disturbing me from my inside. It was to do with the results of my clients. I had imbibed an excellent lesson from my stint with Seb. And that was to maintain some communication with your clients even if you were not professionally associated any more. It could be through social media or a simple text wishing them on occasion. Nothing more. What I observed was a bit discerning. **##ALMOST ALL MY EX CLIENTS HAD REGAINED MOST OF THE WEIGHT THEY HAD LOST.##**

Even in a current lot of clients, what I observed was that the results fell into some distinct categories.

1. Some had absolutely fantastic results. About 60%

2. Some had partial results. About 30%

3. Some were total failures. About 10%

4. **THE CLIENTS WHO REGAINED ALL OR PARTIAL WEIGHT POST THEIR STINT WITH ME WAS A STAGGERING 80%**

This observation number 4 would pose a lot of questions to me.

Why is this happening?

Why can't they maintain it? They have all the knowledge now?

What better help do I give them to hold onto to the progress they made?

I would invariably end up comparing them with myself. I couldn't help myself from doing that. After all, I had lost way higher weight than them, and I was still maintaining it. Then why can't they do the same? This question would never leave me.

I knew my program was meaningless if I cannot bring in a permanent change.

There was a certain degree of self-doubt and fear set in. It would manifest in my self-talk. There was literally too much at stake for me. Had I bitten more than I could chew? This self-talk got louder with time. On the other hand, my seminars were happening on a consistent basis. The capital was flowing in. Discussions to take this to the next level were in their final stages.

I was more or less arriving at the conclusion that people are finding it difficult to lose weight because:

1. **THEY LACK WILL POWER.**
2. **THEY ARE NOT DISCIPLINED.**
3. **THEY ARE NOT FOLLOWING THE PROGRAM MADE FOR THEM.**
4. **THEY ARE ADDICTED TO FOOD.**
5. **THEY DON T WANT TO PUT IN THE HARD YARDS.**
6. **THEY ARE GENETICALLY FAT.**

All the above reasons must be appearing familiar to you. Because this is the narrative around weight loss and the failure to achieve weight loss.

THE TRAINER AND THE TRAINEE ARE BOTH USING THE SAME NARRATIVE.

The trainer uses this to absolve himself from any responsibility because he has taken a fee for his services. Nothing wrong with taking professional charges. But not taking responsibility points towards the integrity of the trainer.

The trainee uses the narrative so that he has an escape from the guilt and shame associated with failing a test. We have been programmed to take weight loss as some sort of test or challenge. So the trainee needs a handy reason to justify his failure. This is how I became a part of the billion-dollar heist around weight loss.

I would conveniently use this narrative as my self talk. "There is only that much I can do after all ", I used to tell myself.

In the midst of this self-talk, it was like a machine type consistency:

Clients kept signing up.

My weekend sojourns to various cities continued.

Life had become a working holiday.

My capital had grown to a healthy level.

I was not too far from becoming a celebrity trainer. Just to give you some food for thought at this point in our conversation, "By the time I reached the end of 2017, I had clients in more than 20 cities in India ". In addition to that, I had scores of clients in **SYDNEY, MELBOURNE, LONDON, FRANKFURT, DUBAI, NAIROBI, SINGA-PORE, DHAKA, KUALA LUMPUR, LAHORE, CAL-IFORNIA, SAN JOSE, DURBAN, COLOMBO, PARIS AND STOCKHOLM.**

I have visited most of these places and conducted workshops. The youngest person I trained was a 16-year-old teenager, and the senior-most person was a spritely 82-year-old. My programs were an instant hit, and the demand for my services was skyrocketing. My calendar was getting full way in advance. The statistics remained more or less the same, and the only bit of stat, which was a constant source of worry for me was that of the percentage of people regaining all or most of their weight.

80%

You would think why the hell am I constantly flashing this 80% figure for you?

I had promised to share all the important aspects of my journey with you at the start of this conversation. So you must be seized of the importance of this question. The answer to the question was **PROFOUND AND THE OUTCOME A WATERSHED MOMENT FOR ME.**

I was riding on a high horse by then. Nothing could go wrong. I was on my way to be the next big thing on the weight loss canvass of the world (there was no harm in thinking like that)—a trainer with international exposure and world-class content. A champagne life and just enormous prospects beckoning.

Let me give you a date for a perspective now.

As mentioned earlier that by the middle of 2018, I had a truly international footprint as far as my business was concerned. And the last client I signed up for weight loss programs was the end of 2018. I have not signed anyone for a weight loss program since then.

Why did I move away from such a successful concept?

Was there an accident or tragic event which made me do that?

Did I suffer from a mental breakdown due to the workload?

Was it too competitive?

Did I stop enjoying it?

Was there any foul play?

Did the market evaporate?

IF IT'S NONE OF THE ABOVE, THEN WHY?

I was committed towards my business, and it was moving in the right direction. All business ventures have their challenges and mine was no different. But no significant dramas. Remember the question sticking to my thoughts.

"why can't people lose weight, and if they do, then why do they regain it?"

I was relentless in my pursuit to find an answer. And I would use an alibi in my self talk to camouflage my inability to find one. The figure of 80% was way too big to ignore or overlook. I knew there was something way more significant than what was evident to my naked eyes or to the knowledge which I had.

AND NO ONE SEEMS TO BE TALKING ABOUT THIS.

It was like a deliberate attempt to hide an uncomfortable truth and jeopardise the **BILLION DOLLAR PIE.** And I was part of that conspiracy. I had become part of a well-oiled machine whose only motive, as its bedrock, was to bandage an issue and actually let the problem fester. The principal was simple :

Grab the issue.

Create a negative narrative around it.

Create fear.

Offer a solution but ensure it never gets solved.

Expand the tribe.

I used words like will power, positivity and motivation liberally. Everyone was using them. All conversations nowadays are around the concept of positivity and negativity. It's like a buzzword. Your social media accounts must be getting inundated with "positive" quotes right from the time you wake up till you sleep. Your WhatsApp feed will be filled with forwards of "ways to lead a better life", cures to the most prominent killer diseases and everything that you can think of. It seems as if the entire world has taken upon itself to rid you of all your issues. I too found myself in the midst of this madness. Despite being a very lite social media user, it was impossible to totally insulate my feeds from that load of crap. It was just irritating, to begin with. But then I started observing **PATTERNS** in this madness.

We are surrounded by a constant barrage of information. Everything around us is geared at catching our attention. Our social media, the television channels, the hoardings on the streets, signages in shops, newspapers, magazines you name it. They want to grab our attention.

AND THERE IS NOTHING BIGGER TO GRAB YOUR ATTENTION THAN FEAR.

On the one hand, you are being sold absolutely unhealthy products like fizzy drinks, preserved synthetic juices, trans-fat-laden snacks, zero nutrition meal substitutes, carcinogenic cooking mediums, magic health portions, chemically manufactured cosmetics, chemical substitutes for sugar, the list is endless. Simultaneously you are offered solutions to the mess your health might be in.

Now just note how this is marketed to you:

- the most popular heroines and models are used to promote these products. The one with the "best complexion" will be used to market facial cosmetics. **YOU ARE SUBTLY MADE TO BELIEVE THAT BEING FAIR IS GOOD.**

- The most well-built actors and models will be used to sell energy drinks. THE SUBTLE **MESSAGE IS THAT YOU WILL BECOME LIKE THEM.**

- The green colour is used extensively in packaging. **YOU HAVE BEEN SUBTLY MADE TO UNDERSTAND**

THAT GREEN MEANS "NATURAL".

- Your favourite actress will be shown choosing to buy particular breakfast cereal. The **SUBTLE MESSAGE HERE IS THAT YOU CAN FEED YOUR FAMILY LIKE YOUR FAVOURITE CELEBRITY.**

- The most popular action heroes will be used to market fizzy drinks. **THE SUBTLE MESSAGE HERE IS THAT ITS COOL TO CONSUME THESE.**

Everything sold is being linked with some celebrity. This clearly impacts our choices. Going to a grocery store, even without you being aware of it, your preferences would have already been made. And this bombardment is incessant and nonstop. So a valid question arising in your thoughts right now will be," how is my weight loss failure linked with the shampoo I bought ?".

(we are very close to answering the 2 questions at the start of this chapter.)

IT ABSOLUTELY IS LINKED, MY FRIEND.

Let me explain this to you. On the one hand, you are constantly bombarded with these images of popular faces consuming certain products. And on the other hand, you are constantly reminded of your poor health by using the same faces.

If you happen to be a person with dark skin, then you will be bombarded with skin lightening solutions because having a lighter skin makes you better . And if you happen to be a fair-skinned person, then you will be bombarded with a skin tanning solution because having darker skin prevents certain types of skin diseases.

The same hero will be shown consuming a particular fizzy drink, and then the same face will be used somewhere else as YOUR HEALTH BENCHMARK. Wow. The same set of faces are used to first get you hooked to some product, which might be absolutely unhealthy, and then those same set of faces are being used to tell you what your health benchmark should be. And it doesn't end here. There are the images used to tell you how inadequate you are and what needs to be done to remove that inadequacy. (**I can actually list out names of celebrities and the products endorsed by them. It will become so clear when you see the pattern. But I am bound by legalities**)

THIS IS CALLED CONSCIOUSNESS HACKING MY FRIEND.

Your entire consciousness, your complete thought processes and your complete mental chemistry have been hacked. It has been hacked to bring your health to where it is now. And it will remain hacked. It might sound ridiculous at first, but think again what I had started sometime back:

YOU GET FAT IN YOUR HEAD. BUT IT SHOWS ON YOUR BODY.

And then comes the billion-dollar industry. It keeps you engaged where the weight shows…your body. But it keeps the issue alive where it started in the first place….

your head.

This was the answer I was searching for. And the moment I understood the link, the entire riddle of "why people find it difficult to lose weight and why they regain it?", had a solution—an answer.

I had inadvertently become a part of that plot to exploit peoples fears and inadequacies. I knew what was missing in the programs being dished out by myself or any other equivalent thing in the market. Everything and everyone was addressing the symptom, which in this case was being overweight. But no one was even glancing at the core of the problem, including myself.

I was pretty crossed with myself for overlooking this important point. How could have I overlooked this when I was myself struggling to lose weight? I knew exactly how one feels from inside when your favourite food item is close to you, and you are trying to lose weight. **It is one thing to deliver sermons and a very different thing when it comes to experiencing it.**

I know you want to pose a question right now. And it would be," when I was in a similar state of my consciousness being hacked, then how come I didn't regain my weight ?"

You are so correct to ask this. And let me tell you how this happened.

For starters, I didn't understand any such concepts of "consciousness hacking". But if we recapitulate our initial conversation, I had mentioned that I have always been a very lite social media user. This was mainly due to me isolating myself from the outside world. I was in Canberra at that time, and my only source of entertainment was the television. And please don't forget that I had piled on oodles of weight during that phase. Remember how I consumed alcohol and junk food sitting in front of the television? But the moment I started working with Seb, I had put all my energies into content research.

Over here, I would like to mention, I was very fortunate that I got introduced to some of the best minds of the world—namely **Dr Joe Dispenza, Dr Bruce Lipton, Mihaly Csikszentmihalyi, Dr Deepak Chopra and Yuval Harari**. There are many more names but the ones mentioned here, stand out for me.

My entire research used to be around the works of these gentlemen. **AND NONE OF THEM WAS A NUTRITIONIST**. I was so desperate to put my life back on rails that I squeezed out the last drop of time by reading what these people had put out. And it was not casual reading. I still have handwritten notes, from that time, of my learnings from the books these gentlemen have published or the talks they have given. So you can say that "I had protected my consciousness from being hacked". It was not by design. But the end result was so. I followed their research and put in practice specific suggestions and routines which acted on the core of my issues.

I will list them out for you shortly. Don't worry.

I was introduced to the **concepts of brain waves and subconscious**. How our brain functions. The function of our senses. The idea of **cellular memory**. The concept of **quantum reality and Neuroplasticity**. All of these are beyond the purview of our present conversation. But extremely vital to understand why and how my entire approach to weight loss changed forever.

There was a complete oversight on my part that I ignored these concepts while I was making personalised programs for people desperate to lose weight. Once I identified the flaw, it did not take much time to reconfigure my entire approach. I could now put scientific reasoning to almost every failure I encountered until that point. More importantly, I could put the reason behind my personal success in a holistic way. It was not just my body I was working on. **I was working on my mind at** the same time. **The change happened** at the **"mind "level**. The physical changes got **firmly anchored** to the mind changes and have become permanent. I wanted the same quality of changes in my clients. Only that would bring in permanent satisfaction to me. Only that would serve my life purpose. The very reason that I gave up a comfortable job in Melbourne was that I was chasing a **"life purpose"**. And if I tried to **WINDOW DRESS** my own purpose, it would leave me a feeling of **guilt and hollowness**. I was not game for that at all. Just the thought that I had become part of an organised loot left me disgusted to the core.

((** **Do you understand now, why I didn't put out a fancy attention-grabbing title to this conversation? Be-**

cause a title anchored to someone's fear will not help me in achieving my life purpose. And that purpose is to help people get a handle on their physical and emotional healths **))

I had to reconfigure this, and I didn't waste any time in doing so. I added some modules in the programs already running for my clients. **I removed any signage** which remotely appeared to be preying upon the vulnerabilities of people. My presentations had a **holistic** approach now. I was laying almost all my focus on the mind part now. Weight loss was just a mention along with a host of other issues. I was convinced that if people are made to understand the core where the problems have their genesis, then people stand an excellent chance of sorting any issue. That includes weight loss. I wanted people to know about the tools used to **HACK THEIR CONSCIOUSNESS**. The same tools could be used to bring about changes at the core level. It is all in the brain waves.

If I want you to remember just ONE CONCEPT from this entire conversation, then that is the concept of brain waves.

Yes. This is **"WHERE ANGELS CONSPIRE".**

If we understand the working of our brain, we will never allow it to be hacked by anyone.

Let me list out a few interesting facts about our bodies. All this information is available in the public domain. It is not classified.

- The fastest supercomputer in the world is supposedly in China. Its name is Tianhe-2. Its processing speed is 54.902 petaflops. One petaflop is a quadrillion floating-point calculations per second (one quadrillion is a thousand trillion). In comparison, the human brain is postulated to have a processing speed of 1 exaflop. That is a billion billion calculations per second. In 2014, some researchers in Japan tried to match the processing power of **1% of the human brain in one second**. It took the 4th fastest computer of that time, named the K computer, **40 minutes** to match that.

- An adult human body has anything between 50-100 trillion cells. Each cell has DNA inside the nucleus. If we open up a cell and unwrap the DNA, then the DNA strand would measure 5 feet. If we take out all the DNA from all those cells and string them together, then that string would make 150 round trips to the sun.

- In about 6 months, 99% of human cells are replaced by brand new cells.

- Our heart circulates the entire blood about 1000 times each day.

- The total length of the blood vessels in humans is about 100,000 km.

- Our bones are 4 times stronger than concrete.

- The human brain has memory capacity in excess of 4 terabytes of a hard drive.

- Nerve impulses from the brain move at a speed of 274 km/hr.

- About 100,000 chemical reactions occur in the human brain every second.

- A human eye can distinguish 10 million different colours.

I just listed out a few popular ones. But so often we forget all this. And it's mainly due to the negative narrative being peddled around us 24x7.

It will not add to the BILLION DOLLAR HEIST if you are reminded of your greatness. So it is a multi-pronged strategy. it's simple :

KEEP THEM IN A STATE OF FEAR AND KEEP REINFORCING THOSE FEARS.

And this is not limited to weight loss. I have deliberately picked this topic to initiate a conversation. The entire narrative around us is "**DEEPLY ANCHORED TO HARNESS THE FEARS OF THE MASSES**". What might appear as a harmless promotion of a product might be ushering you towards something else? Images and visuals are bombarded at us to hack our consciousness.

Remember the question I had asked in the initial part of our conversation regarding Obama. It works exactly in that way—our brain functions on images. The words you read are also images. The words you hear are matched to images. The aromas you detect are attached to some image. And then these images are used to arrive at a meaning. So a popular actor or model who has enacted as a saintly character, in some television serial or movie, when appears in promotion of a "packaged juice" brand, will be interpreted by your brain as," this is good for me because a good man has it". I hope you are now able to find the link between the images used to sell you a shampoo and your weight gain.

I was extremely cognizant of this during my own struggles with my issues. And I used to stay away from all of this. I did not understand the implications of me staying away from this audiovisual brain hacking. But I just stayed away. It was only when I was struggling to find the solution to the "80%" failure rate that the mind-body connect dawned on me. It was never the same for me after that. My entire focus and strategy shifted to explain this connection. To my pleasant surprise, there were far more takers for this concept. People were inquisitive. They were genuinely interested to learn about this. It was easier for them to understand the concept of consciousness hacking. I used to carry with me samples of packed products to my shows. I used to record the commercials and run them again as part of my presentation. I made people **read labels** on the so-called **"healthy products".** The entire flavour of the approach became **EXPERIENTIAL.** It was all about touch feel see and smell. I started cataloguing the contents of many popular products. I would then research those contents and put the findings in a mail form and send it to all my clients—both past and present. People latched onto this genre of information. Their grocery checklists changed. Their routines changed. Their healths became better.

WEIGHT LOSS WAS NOW A BYPRODUCT. NOT AN END PRODUCT.

There is a vast qualitative difference in the statement. Let me explain.

An "end product" is the desired result of a process. Like the end product of a car assembly line will be a fully functional car.

A "byproduct" is a product which gets obtained during the process of getting the main product. So in a car assembly line, one of the byproducts will be metal scrap. No doubt that the byproduct is useful in deciding the final price of the product, in this case, a car, but the fact remains that metal scrap is a byproduct of the process which produces cars.

NOW ASK THIS QUESTION TO YOURSELF

Will you put in a car assembly line in place so that you can get scrap metal???

This is exactly what we do. **We think that the byproduct is the main product.** And this is due to the consciousness hacking happening all the time. We are chasing a byproduct called weight loss.

So what should be the main product in our conversation?

THE MAIN PRODUCT IS OUR SUBCONSCIOUS.

If we work towards reprogramming our subconscious, it will change everything within you. Weight loss will happen automatically.

This conversation is beginning to get a bit serious and technical from here. I will make an attempt to explain this core concept in straightforward words. The complete information is available easily on the net, and it is fascinating. I will refrain from using any complicated terminology or concepts. We will stick to some fundamental concepts to make this learning enjoyable. Once you get a grip of the core of the concept, then you can start investing your time to enhance your learnings. This is precisely what I did. Let's begin.

For that, we have to go back to the time you were just born. We will need to learn about brain waves. Have a look at the simple brain wave chart below.

BETA BRAINWAVES.

ALPHA BRAINWAVES.

THETA BRAINWAVES.

DELTA BRAINWAVES.

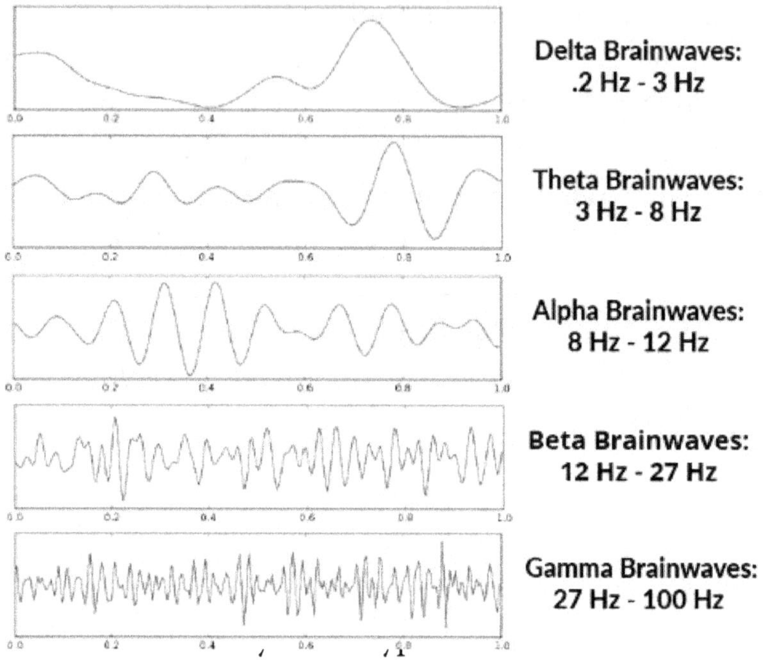

gamma, lambda and epsilon. But the above 4 are what we need to understand in the context of our conversation. All these waves have a specific frequency. Brain waves, in simple terms, are signatures of your brain activity. These are easily measured using an **EEG machine (electroencephalogram)**. Just by looking at the frequencies, you will see that higher frequencies are related to higher brain activity. Like right now, you are in the Beta Zone. This zone is linked with your alertness and is experienced during your wakeup state. You stay in this zone all day as you go about your daily routine.

The next zone is the Alpha zone. This is linked with lower brain activity. Like when you are relaxing or when you want to go to sleep. The alertness levels drop here. But you are still fully awake. It's the daydreaming zone.

Then we have the Theta zone. This is when you start loosing your conscious state. It's sort of a hypnogogic state. Your body becomes very relaxed. Muscles lose their tautness. Your alertness drops completely. Your "mind" is totally open to suggestions and ideas. You don't have control over your body. It starts feeling like jelly.

The last zone is the Delta zone. This is total sleep zone. You lose all your conscious state.

NOTE: there are many more brain waves, and all this information is available in the public domain. You don't need a licence to access this. The knowledge extracted from that information is being used by **multinationals, broadcasters, social media platforms, advertising agencies, wellness industry, food companies, tobacco companies, breweries, the fashion industry and entertainment industry**, to hack into your consciousness. Let's learn how.

Now take a look at this BELL CURVE as shown in the diagram.

1. BETA 7

2. ALPHA 6

3. THETA 5

4. DELTA

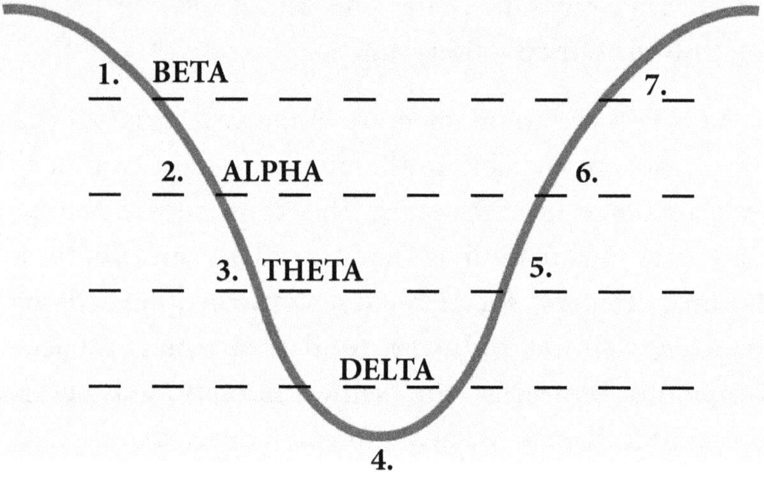

This bell curve depicts the 24-hour brain activity of a normal human being. Let's decode this in simple terms.

1. **BETA.** You are fully awake and going about your daily routine. Eating, driving, writing, thinking, planning, talking, crossing the road, having sex, arguing, gymming, surfing your social media feeds, watching television and just about everything. **YOU ARE FULLY CONSCIOUS AND ALERT IN THIS STATE.** It's an essential state for you to function during the day and lead your life.

2. **ALPHA.** You have retired after your dinner and are reading a book or watching television or going

through your social media feed and preparing to fall asleep. It's a very relaxed mode, and your body relaxes. Your senses are still active, but they are not that acute now. You could be in your own thoughts. But you are still awake.

3. **THETA.** Your alertness levels drop drastically. You are almost asleep but still just awake. The body feels like jelly.

4. **DELTA.** You are in a deep sleep. You have no sensation of your body now.

Now, this was sort of repeated.

Relax my friend. Let's look at the next few numbers (5, 6 and 7)

5. **THETA.** You have slept through the nite, and your body clock now clicks in to wake you up. The brain activity starts going up. You get out of the deep sleep state back into the THETA state. You are not yet awake. It's that same hypnogogic state. The body is like jelly. You are on your way to wake up.

6. **ALPHA.** You can now make out some sensations around you like sounds, smell and visuals. You are awake. You have complete control over your body. The brain is still relaxed after a restful nite (hopefully). You are fully awake but still in a relaxed mode.

7. **BETA.** You are back to your daily routine.

This bell curve is repeated each day of your life. From the time you were born till the last day of your life. This is pure science, and there is no religious or spiritual connotation to this. The only thing that differs in this curve, from the time you were born till the end of your life, is the time you spend in those zones at various stages of your life. Let me elaborate.

At birth, your brain spent most of its time in the delta and theta zones. Delta mainly. (have you noticed that newborns are sleeping most the time.) As you started growing, you spent more and more time in the theta zone. The time spent in beta and Alpha is minimal. Within the first few months of your life, you start spending a little more time in the alpha and beta zones. But the time spent in Theta and Delta outstrips the time spent in the other two zones.

What is the implication of this? This is where all the action is happening. And you just thought that what was the big deal in this seemingly innocuous happening.

Think again.

At the time of your birth, there are practically zero levels of conscious behaviour. Everything is a brand new input for the infant. Each input gets accepted without any question being asked. Our questions are a product of our conscious mind. At birth, there is none of it. Everything coming our way gets embedded into the subconscious part of our mind.

Neuroscience and psychology have now concluded that almost 80% of your **subconscious programming** happens within the time frame of your **birth and 9-10 years** of your life. This is where your choices, habits, temperament, leanings, likes and dislikes are formed. This part of your mind controls your complete life. Subconscious is not a physical part of the brain.

It is a program which resides in a part of the brain known as the "cerebellum ".

Feeling a bit confused? I know how your **reasoning mind, "the conscious mind",** will not let you accept this. Let me give you a modern analogy here.

Say you take a nonstop flight from Melbourne to Delhi. The approximate time of this flight time is about 12 hours. So you are a passenger in a 12-hour flight. And if its a flight then obviously it's being flown by a team of pilots. Correct?

It's not exactly like that. Yes, there is a team of pilots. But for close to 11 hours of that flight time of 12 hours, the aircraft is being flown by a **software program called the "autopilot ".**

Yes, you heard it right. For 11 hours of the total flight time, your aircraft is not being manually controlled. The autopilot is an extremely sophisticated software program which factors in thousands of factors at the same time and keeps the plane on track to its final destination. While you were having a polite conversation with a co-passenger over a drink, your flight was being run by a program. The pilots are always there, but their role is limited to certain situations only.

Your subconscious is a similar program, albeit far more sophisticated, on which you run your life. At birth, there is no program in the subconscious. It gets formed as you start spending some time in the Beta, Alpha and Theta zones. Your **programmers** at that time are your **parents, family, neighbours and family friends.** Your brain just catches each and every input coming your way. That input could be of aromas, tastes, colours, religious leanings, political choices, spoken language, cultural preferences, food choices and everything you can imagine. And because :

1. There is no program existing in your subconscious at birth and

2. You spend most of the time in Alpha, Theta and Delta zones (the time from birth till a few years)

Each and every input becomes part of the subconscious program. This programming keeps happening incessantly until the ages of about 9-10 years. It is said that it could be as much as 80% by the time you are 10 years and 95% by the time you are 35 years. These numbers are not a creation of my imagination. These are a result of extensive scientific and psychological research of the past 100 years done by researchers and scientists.

So here comes the exciting part.

Your mental programming is almost 95% complete by the time you are 35-year-old adult, and now you want to change some aspect of your personality. It could be your :

- Food habits.
- Spending habits.
- Temperament issues such as anger.
- Relationship issues.

- Sexual habits.
- Financial issues.
- Religious or spiritual orientations.

IT APPEARS TO BE AN IMPOSSIBLE TASK.

My friend the program running your life will not let you deviate from the choices and inputs which formed the basis of that program. On a lighter note, "the autopilot will ensure that you reach Delhi on that flight which you embarked on from Melbourne."

If you have grown up with particular food and eating habits, then it seems impossible to change those habits. **It's not a coincidence that overweight parents have overweight children**. Those children will grow up as overweight adults and have children who will get overweight. Then we hear the most common explanations to this like:

- **It runs in my family**
- **I have tried so hard but failed.**
- **I have low will power.**
- **This is my destiny.**

"IT IS NOT YOUR DESTINY, MY FRIEND."

Mark my words. Make a note of them. What you call as your "destiny", is the net result of the choices you make in every moment of your living life. And these choices are governed by the program which runs in the background. That program is called the subconscious and has a signature called "brain waves". If you take deliberate steps in understanding these waves, then a pathway to your subconscious opens up. Once you have that pathway, then you will be able to "reprogram your subconscious". Words like **impossible, destiny, fate, addictions, willpower and motivation** will lose their present meaning to you.

The situation is crystal clear here. Either you own your brain waves, or the entire world is out there to capture them. There are many more contours and shades to this concept of "subconscious "which I have not brought up in this conversation. I have deliberately kept it to the most simplistic level for ease of understanding. There is a lot of noise about concepts such as karma, past life, chakras, tantra, mantra, cosmic unity etc. All of these are fantastic concepts, and there is a lot of research happening about them. I am myself investing a lot of my time on a few of these. But let's not bring them up here. That can happen over another conversation, at another time. I "promise that".

We initiated this conversation around my state and how I succeeded in shedding oodles of weight and then kept it away. As I mentioned earlier, the weight gain happened in my head first, and then it started showing on my body. The information on weight gain was riding on my brain waves.

Just like the way your favourite song rides on some radio waves. The song is not inside the radio. The radio has a receiver which captures those radio waves and transforms those waves to sound waves which you call "a song". The sound waves from the radio set fall on your eardrums.

They get converted to a wave pattern which your brain captures and gives it a meaning. Just imagine the amount of technology at work in a simple event of you listening to a song.

It doesn't end here. Attached to the song could be some memories. And attached to those memories are feelings. **Thoughts are for your mind. Feelings are for your body**. The messenger boys between your mind and body are chemicals we call "hormones". A good memory will activate a different set of chemicals from that of a bad memory. Your body is simply responding to these chemical stimulations. It all starts with a wave.

Tell me something here before we proceed. Have you noticed how you feel in your body when you get angry at someone? The anger in your brain is transmitted to your body. In mild anger response, you could feel some warmth all over your body, there will be a slight increase in your heart rate and your entire focus shifts to the issue which created the issue. In extreme cases of anger, your body will experience shivering and heart rates become very high. Each thought has to translate into a feeling. **THIS IS MIND AND BODY UNITY**. Similarly, a happy thought translates into a different body response.

Your body is merely responding to a particular thought at all times.

Will, it be fair to ask then," any addiction is just a body response to a brain wave?". The answer is yes.

You must have heard the term "withdrawal symptoms". This is your body sending signals in the reverse direction to the brain to abandon a new behaviour it might be attempting to follow. Most likely, you will fail to install that new behaviour. You have access to a mere 5% of your consciousness, and you are trying to pit it against 95% of your consciousness which is already programmed and will not budge. There is nothing like a GOOD OR BAD subconscious. It is just a program which controls your habits and behaviour. Non-vegetarian struggles to understand that how could anyone survive without meat. Vegetarian struggles to understand that how can anyone consume an animal. I am not getting into the debate about what is better. I just want you to realise that the beliefs and habits installed in the subconscious mind will not allow you to drift away from those very beliefs and practices. **"the subconscious is a perfect autopilot"**.

Do you understand why is it impossible to follow a new diet even when you know that the same diet can help you lose weight?

So what do we do now?

Your life is running on a program which will not let you change to a new scheme of things. So is there any point to even try to "change ?"

Something which happened in the period between your birth and till about 10 years of your life, how can you undo that programming now?

And the world has not yet seen a **TIME MACHINE WHICH CAN TAKE ME BACK TO MY BIRTH**.

(just trying to bring in some humour my friend)

Here is where **NEUROSCIENCE** comes to our aid.

The world has seen an absolute exponential growth in the fields of Neuroscience, pharmacology, technology and psychology in the last 3 decades. Our understanding of the functioning of the human brain has grown by leaps and bounds in this time period. Brain imaging technology has actually provided us with tools which give us an opportunity to "peek into the secret world of the human brain." It has given us some glimpses of the playfield "**WHERE ANGELS CONSPIRE**".

It might sound metaphoric.

But it is not. Let me explain.

We have grown up listening to many stories, told to us by our elders. Those stories were mainly about kings and queens or mythological beings. The word "angel" brings out an image of some mystical creature who is draped in white robes, mist-like, winged and riding a white unicorn. The picture depends upon the bedtime stories we were told as children (programming the subconscious again. In my case, it used to be a bearded man). Those angels had the powers to get us anything. They had the capabilities of curing us of disease. If we made them happy, then they could reverse any adverse situation. They came only at night after we sleep. Those angels were the "good be-

ings" sent to vanquish the "evil beings". They were not visible to the naked eyes.

All cultures, regardless of where that culture flourished on the planet, are replete with the concept of angels and fairies. And these stories were told to children at bedtime. The child would fall asleep while listening to such accounts.

What used to be a ritual passed from one generation to the next, has now become a multi-billion dollar business of bedtime storybooks. The routine is "intact". I can bet, here, that 99% of adults don't have a clue to the reason for this well-entrenched ritual. I have asked this question to thousands of people. The most common response is that it helps children fall asleep. Of course, they fall asleep. They will fall asleep even if you don't tell them a bedtime story. Even you fall asleep. No one comes to tell you a bedtime story. Isn't it ???? ##

Then why this ritual. I request you go through this last bit of our conversation again. (Yes, I insist with folded hands. Just the bit marked between ## symbols).

Let me unzip the deep neuroscience hidden in this seemingly innocent ritual. Let's dissect each bit :

- bedtime stories being told only to young children. **SUBCONSCIOUS PROGRAMMING POSSIBLE ONLY IN CHILDREN.**

- Those angels are capable of curing any diseases. **THE HUMAN GROWTH HORMONE IS RELEASED ONLY WHEN YOU ARE IN DEEP SLEEP. DELTA**

ZONE.

- Happy angels can reverse any situation. **INSTALLING BETTER BELIEFS. AGAIN SUBCONSCIOUS PROGRAMMING.**

- Angels not visible to anyone with naked eyes and visit only during sleep. **ALLUDING TO THE BRAINWAVES DURING THE SLEEPING TIME.**

It is nothing less than magical how the different cultures had the same understanding of the subconscious and the importance of installing the right beliefs (programs) at the right time. Our minds are like a blank slate at birth. What we write on that slate is what determines our entire lives. Those bedtime stories were the magical tools with which beliefs were installed on the blank subconscious.

The last 50 years have seen a serious erosion of such potent rituals. We still have bedtime rituals. Stories for children have been replaced by television sops. It's common to fall asleep with the television remote in our hand or the mobile dropping on our chests. What's the big deal in this, you must be thinking.

My friend it's not about a deal. You get an opportunity to "REPROGRAM THE SUBCONSCIOUS" during your sleep not once, but twice. You get this divine opportunity to scrub the programs sitting in your subconscious and replacing them with brand new beliefs (programs). These new belief systems will lead to new choices. The new choices will lead to new and better behaviours. All these will start translating into desired results. **"The Angels are your brain waves in a very specific frequency**

window ". That window opens for a short duration twice, during each sleep cycle. **That window is when you transition from the Alpha to the Theta state and from the Theta to the Alpha state.**

All this knowledge is now available thanks to brain imaging techniques and neurosciences. The bell curve is a result of that knowledge. We are living in an era of human history where we can choose to use this knowledge and advancements either to become what we "want to" or allow someone else to use it against us. We can choose to guard and nurture our brain waves or let them be abused and deformed by external forces.

The greatest ever scientist to have walked this planet, **Albert Einstein,** harnessed this concept to arrive at some of the most profound theories. **Thomas Edison** made most of his discoveries by leveraging these brain wave states. **Nicola Tesla** was a master of his brain waves. Some of the best musical creations have happened in the midst of these brain waves. The **deepest** and the most **profound spiritual wisdom** has been the outcome of saints and mystics remaining immersed in these brainwave states.

The beauty of all of this is that there is an equal opportunity for every human to master these brain waves states. No one is excused from that opportunity. It's only a matter of our personal choices.

The conversation commenced around a weight loss journey. And it has now become a journey of reprogramming your destiny. The endeavours of everyone could be diverse. Someone could be looking for the elusive **weight loss trick**, someone could be wanting to break the chain of **failed relationships**, someone else could be stuck in a cyclic **financial mess**. Whatever the issue might be, the solution starts with your subconscious mind. Your subconscious mind will keep you in the state from which it was formed. Have you noticed a few facts as stated :

> » rich children get richer.
> » children whose parents are alcoholics or into substance abuse, end up being the same.
> » not so well off people winning huge lotteries generally lose all the winnings within the first few years.
> » children of overweight parents generally will be overweight.
> » children from broken homes will generally have relationship issues as adults.

It's all due to the background program, the inner self-talk which decides what your life is going to be. Remember how I mentioned the "soft small voice" inside me during the phase when I was really struggling with my issues. That small voice is present in everyone. We have to create silence to connect with it.

We will now proceed to have a peep into that elusive window where we get that opportunity to reprogram our subconscious. It's the window where you get the chance to **mimic divinity**. The window "**Where Angels Conspire** ".

"Happiness is a choice, not a result. Nothing will make you happy unless you choose to be happy. No person will make you happy unless you decide to be happy. Your Happiness never comes to you. It comes from within you"

BUDDHA.

"The time is always right to do what is right"

MARTIN LUTHER KING Jr.

CHAPTER SEVEN

THE WINDOW TO THE DEVINE PLAYFIELDS

We have, indeed, travelled a lot of distance in our conversation. Let me unfold the science behind this concept of brain waves. We will look at both the diagrams in conjunction over here. The reason I brought up the idea of bedtime stories was singularly scientific. Read the next few sentences carefully.

A thought captured during the transition from the Beta state into the Alpha state and from the Alpha state into the Theta state…will remain captive and alive in your subconscious. Because after the Theta state, you will get into a deep state of sleep called the Delta state. The window of opportunity opens for a concise duration when you transition from Alpha to Theta. As you observe the bell curve, the window opens twice during your sleep cycle.

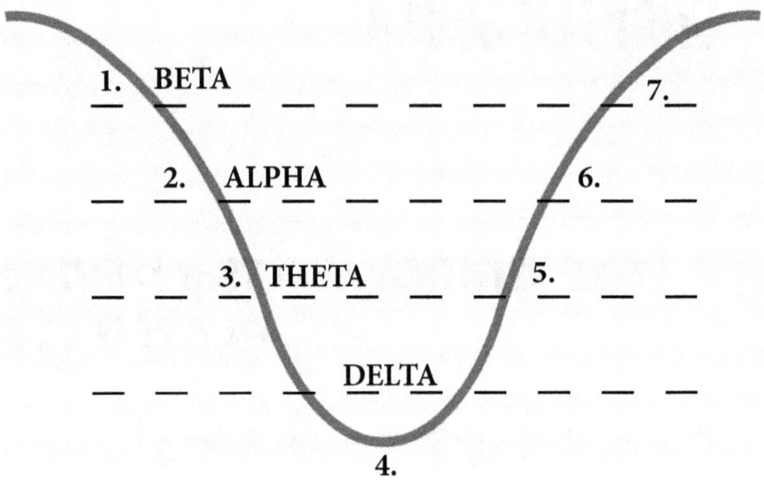

1. What do I mean when I state that "a thought being captured ".

All through our day, we are continually getting inputs through our conscious mind, and we are responding to those inputs based on our beliefs in the subconscious mind. So each and every thought is being given a response. A thought and a response complete the circuit. Just at that moment of us loosing our conscious state, the last thought goes into the subconscious to get a response. But it can't escape as the window gets shut and the circuit can't be completed. That thought is now in a **"captured state ".**

2. So what happens when a thought is captured in the subconscious?

Your subconscious is just a recorder of any input that falls on your conscious mind. If any input reaches you, it is captured by your subconscious mind. No questions are asked. All your questions arise due to your conscious mind. Your conscious mind is the analytical mind. The subconscious mind is your data bank. And it's a huge data bank. Some calculations have projected a mind-numbing figure. Researchers say that by the time a human reaches the age of 21 years, the subconscious mind has stored information equivalent to the combined knowledge of **100 Encyclopaedia Britannica**. And this is a non-stop process going on throughout your life. The processing power of the subconscious mind is estimated at about 20,000,000 bits per second.

In comparison, our conscious mind, which resides in the neocortex region of our brain, has a processing capacity of about 40 bits per second. So the processing power of your subconscious mind is 500,000 times that of your conscious mind. Due to the limited processing capacity of the conscious mind, we register and analyse only a fraction of those inputs. But everything gets recorded in the subconscious. Now, as we are falling asleep, the final thoughts or inputs entering our conscious mind get trapped in the subconscious mind. The window between the conscious mind and the subconscious mind shuts the moment you slip into the Delta zone(deep sleep). The conscious mind is also sleeping (shut down) at this time.

BUT NOT YOUR SUBCONSCIOUS MIND. IT NEVER SLEEPS. All your internal body functions are controlled by the subconscious mind. Can you stop your heart from beating? Do you control what happens to the food after you eat it? Do you even think about your breathing at any given time of the day or night? Your subconscious keeps everything going. (this part of the subconscious gets formed from before you were born. It's an evolutionary chain of events. We are born with a bit of the subconscious already programmed. Our discussion falls outside the purview of those concepts)

The job of the subconscious mind is to match any input (thought) with the stored information and provide an output (solution) for the conscious mind. As the window between the two is shut, while you are in a deep sleep, and no fresh input is coming from the conscious mind, the subconscious mind keeps processing the same information. The subconscious does not ask any questions. It just tries to match a piece of information with the data stored and provide a solution.

NOW COMES THE CRITICAL PART

Any input (a thought) will be matched with the already stored information (a response). This information could be beliefs, prejudices, choices and biases. These responses were formed in the first few years of your life (remember the phase where your subconscious was blank and was getting programmed). It's all good as long as that thought matches with a stored response. But in the event of a thought not finding a match in the stored data bank of reactions, **"HOUSTON WE HAVE A PROBLEM"**. The subconscious reads this as an intrusion. And it tries to remind you to change that thought. But you are sleeping (the conscious mind is unresponsive). The poor subconscious mind has to deal with this situation all night. It is uncomfortable with this situation. It will use all its might to find a match to this thought and provide a solution (a response).

THE RULE is that a new thought will only match with a new response.

At first, it will be challenging for the subconscious to find the exact match. It will let you know of its annoyance by throwing at you feelings such as cravings. In extreme cases, your body will also join the subconscious by showing signs of withdrawal symptoms. It could be cramps, palpitations, sweating, or anything physical which will make you feel that the pain and discomfort to you are being caused by the "NEW THING" that you are trying to do. So don't be surprised at the cravings for your favourite snack within the first few hours of you decide to stop consuming it. How many times have you experienced the amplified urge of doing the very thing which you want to stop doing?

Let me share some everyday experiences to explain this mysterious way of working of the subconscious.

*Have you experienced a situation when you want to hum a particular song but are getting confused with the music and lyrics. Even after trying hard, you can't get it. But the thought kept on going in your mind even while you are about to hit the bed. You try once last time but still don't get it. Then you just slip into your sleep. Next morning you wake up, and you are singing the song like a nightingale.

From where did you get this? Your subconscious went through all the data and pops it out at the first opportunity it gets.

That first opportunity is the when you are transitioning from the theta to alpha brain wave state. The window opens again for a short time when you are waking up. (refer to the bell curve diagram)

- You have been trying to find some solution for your office work. Despite your best efforts and the knowledge, it eludes you. Something doesn't seem to be in place or is missing. But you keep trying, and still, it eludes you, and you fall asleep still trying to find a solution. You wake up in the morning with the answer in your mind. You just realised that you were overlooking something distinct or a new way appeared as a solution.

- You need some cash. So you find the nearest ATM. You insert your card into the machine and try to remember your password. Somehow you get confused with the different passwords for different things that you have created. You simply can't get it. Your fingers are just over the keypad, and you are still thinking about the numbers. Then suddenly you observe that the fingers seem to know your password. They fall on the exact sequence. This is your body memory. When you do something over and over again, the memory gets entrenched in that body part.

- You are driving to work. Your favourite song is playing in the car music system. You are in thoughts about some meeting or some issue or a project or anything else. You are completely lost in your thoughts. Suddenly your thought chain is broken by a horn or something, and you realise that you have almost reached the office without remembering anything while you were driving. This was your subconscious navigating for you from the stored data bank and the communication channels it has between itself and your entire body.

There are innumerable examples of the types I just mentioned. What I wanted to illustrate is that there is a much bigger and powerful mind running behind the scene of your conscious mind. You simply can't bring in a change by using your conscious mind. The core of the issue is in the subconscious. If you address the issue where it resides, only then will you be able to change behaviour.

The entire wellness industry, in particular the weight loss industry, is giving you a solution which uses your conscious mind.

THEY KNOW IT VERY WELL THAT IT IS DOOMED FOR FAILURE.

The approach is window dressed by using fancy names, sexy looking models, reminding you of some elusive dream, harnessing your fears and the most important, hacking your consciousness by manipulating the brain wave states. I have mentioned this term" consciousness hacking" a several times till now. I will list out shortly the exact sequence of how it is done with you. I will stick to our topic of conversation of weight loss in doing so. Just be patient.

Going back to the subconscious, what you must have realised is where the problem actually resides. The reason you have not been able to overcome a particular issue is not that you have the weak will power or that you are not motivated or that it's your destiny. The primary reason is that you have been trying to change something superficially by using the conscious mind. While the problem is deeply embedded in your subconscious. A simple ray diagram will explain this:

IDENTIFY THE ISSUE>> LIST OUT THE BEHAVIOURS SUPPORTING THE ISSUE>> LIST THE THOUGHTS LINKED WITH THIS BEHAVIOUR>> LETS PLAN NOW.

This part of our work is key to changed behaviour.

There are millions of books and sites on weight loss. There are millions of motivational quotes encircling everyone. There are hundreds of motivational speakers in each city. **BUT THE WORLD IS STILL STRUGGLING WITH OBESITY.** In fact, it's getting worse by the day. Once you list out the behaviour you want to change and the thoughts supporting that behaviour, only then you will be able to replace those behaviours. These behaviours are linked with the beliefs which sit as programs in your subconscious mind. It's effortless to change or plant beliefs in children. Its a cakewalk. That's why the first 10 years are the most critical years of your life. Here, we might be attempting to undo the damage caused during that phase. Keep another point in mind. The subconscious just understands **images and feelings**. Let me explain this with a simple example. Say you want to quit smoking. The thought and desire most people have are:

"I WANT TO QUIT SMOKING ".

Look at the words just mentioned.

The subconscious understands only one word or a part of it. Smoking. It will match this word with images of you or someone smoking. Everything else makes no sense to the subconscious. Remember how I mentioned that everything is stored in the memory bank in the form of images. Even verbs (actions) are stored as images. So when you say "I want to quit smoking", the image which pulls up in the subconscious is of you or someone else smoking. The subconscious will do everything to support this action. So instead of quitting, you will get cravings and withdrawal. And universally people link this to lack of will power.

An alternate for the above statement," I want to quit smoking", can be a statement like **"I have fantastic health "**. Along with this statement, if you imagine an image of yourself with optimum health and eating good food, the subconscious will start working to match that image.

There is no mention of smoking here. But what we are mentioning is the result of quitting smoking. **"HEALTHY"**. Now the subconscious will start matching this word with the stored images in its data bank.

So will this happen over nite? The answer is "A BIG BIG NO".

Please don't have a panacea that taming the subconscious is an over nite job. It's the most powerful piece of software ever created. Each individual has unique software. The software updates and evolves on its own. The combined knowledge and expertise, of the most brilliant minds, is just beginning to understand small bits and pieces of this program.

If you want to attempt to give a number to this intelligence then try this for me please: get a sandwich. Give half of it to your pet and consume the other half. The sandwich becomes "you" when it goes inside you. And it becomes your "pet" when it goes inside your pet. We are living in a computer age where we understand words as "input" and "output". If the sandwich is an input, then how can it have two different outputs. Not convinced yet?

Let's take it a step further. Let's divide the same sandwich between the two of us. We both are humans. But the sandwich becomes me when it goes inside me, and it becomes you when it goes inside you. Still a bit doubtful?

Let's crank this up a bit more. Let's order for some fruits, cakes and coffee. Let's consume them. Different inputs. Same computer. Same result. Anything which goes inside you becomes you. And the same things when going inside me become me.

You are dealing with a beast of a program with infinite potency. That program is unique to your pet, yourself and me. Anything which goes inside us becomes us. ***The food you eat and the thoughts you generate, all become you.***

Do you know the best part of this? This beast is your friend. It's your protector. It's childlike, and It understands bedtime tales. The language of the subconscious is images. These images ride on the thoughts you generate.

There is a way to approach the subconscious mind. If you approach it with your conscious mind (your ego lives in the conscious mind), then you will fail. That's a certainty. You will think that it is possible. You might get some small results. But they will never be permanent. You need to be patient when you are trying to implant a new thought or belief in your subconscious mind. Harnessing the brain waves is critical.

From here, we will discuss some strategies to bring about permanent changes in our beliefs and the behaviours emanating due to those beliefs. No one is an authority in this concept of "subconscious reprogramming". There are cryptic notes on the subject, dating thousands of years. It is abundantly apparent that there was extensive research on the topic in various civilisations. Just as more and more evidence is presenting itself through brain imaging techniques and neurosciences, modern science has started embracing those ancient theories. It is not surprising at all to encounter top-notch scientists using spiritual terminologies and examples during presentations. I love one of the quotes by Albert Einstein on the subject.

"When you examine the lives of the most influential people who have ever walked amongst us, you discover one thread that winds through them all. They have been aligned first with their spiritual nature and only then with their physical selves. "

We can choose to ignore these profound learnings, or we can want to rewrite our stories. The same knowledge is used to hack into your consciousness.

"Never say 'No', never say 'I cannot', for you are infinite. All the power is within you. You can do anything."

SWAMI VIVEKANANDA.

"The intuitive mind is a sacred gift, and the rational mind is the faithful servant. We have created a society that honours the servant and has forgotten the gift"

ALBERT EINSTEIN

CHAPTER EIGHT

REPROGRAMMING THE SUBCONSCIOUS TO SHED SOME WEIGHT

WITNESSING THE ANGELS CONSPIRING

Before we forget, all this was happening while I was in Goa. I had understood the reason why the change in my weight was permanent and why the same permanency was not happening in the case of my clients. My change had occurred at the core level, my subconscious. While my entire strategy with my clients was centred around the physicality, the conscious mind. It was convenient for me to assign the failure of my clients to excuses like lack of will power, motivation and discipline. But the figure of 80% failure rate was way too much for my subconscious to be comfortable with. It dawned upon me that I had become an accessory to the global heist of milking peoples fears and vulnerabilities. **This was not my "purpose of life** "in the first place. I used to feel happy when I could help someone lose weight. And that happiness was a shared feeling. The absence of that feeling was taking me away from my purpose. I knew this was extremely important for me if I wanted to continue doing this.

Something important that I kept doing all these years was to continually upgrade my knowledge of nutrition, biomechanics, neuroscience and psychology. Just to give you an idea about this, I would invest a minimum of 6 hours a day in reading and making notes. The content was not necessarily about weight loss. It would be about energy systems, quantum reality, sound therapies, Ayurveda, yoga, metacognition, flow states, 3rd eye and brain waves states. I had accumulated a lot of content. **It was now just about marrying this with weight loss and wellness**. And I did exactly like that.

I stopped chasing numbers. I had figured out that this chase was the culprit in my becoming an accessory in a global heist. I altered the content of my seminars which were in line with the concept of "**mind-body unity**".

What I will share with you, now, is that same approach. The attendance of my seminars dropped initially. But it was a very temporary phase. These seminars were more to explain the mind-body connect and less about weight loss. I was aware that my entire business model was dependant upon "number of people signing up ". The falling numbers did not deter me one bit. Because the venture was initiated to experience happiness in what I was doing. Nothing else. I had this calming feeling inside me that I had course-corrected myself and returned to my purpose.

I have explained, in some detail, about food, nutrition, weight gain, my personal journey, the psychology behind weight loss, the failures, brain wave states, conscious and subconscious mind. Each of the above can be a totally independent conversation by themselves. My attempt is to condense and compress these concepts to a volume which is helpful to you or anyone else. By no means is this the **"HOLY GRAIL OF WEIGHT LOSS"**. It is and will remain one of the many pathways to good overall health. It should be helpful in making you understand one primary link. The link between mind and body. If you can acknowledge the existence of that link, you will be in a position to change anything around yourself. It could be your:

- **Health issues.**
- **Relationship issues.**
- **Learning issues.**
- **Financial issues.**
- **Spiritual issues.**
- **Professional issues.**

All the above are interlinked somewhere in your core. If any of the above gets disturbed, individually, the impact is felt in all of them. For example, A financial issue has the capacity to impact your relationships. That, in turn, can affect your health and profession. I am not alluding to the daily challenges we face. That's part of life. I am pointing towards any issue which persists for an extended period. My current workshops and training are around the overall state of an individual. That individual could be a person or a business entity.

I will separate out all the points we have discussed until now. It's important that we have a well-structured document readily available for any future reference. This is the EXACT strategy I use to date. The results are permanent. Let's have a look at them.

- **Acknowledgement.**
- **Why and how did I gain weight?**
- **Why do I want to lose weight?**
- **Target weight and target date.**
- **What's the plan?.**

These are the pointers from where we start. Let us expand each one of these.

ACKNOWLEDGEMENT

This is the starting point in your quest to losing weight. Self-denial is the biggest hurdle. Being overweight is a physical condition. Self-denial is a psychological condition. It is the self-talk and creates a toxic web around you. Remember one thing very clearly. FAT is not profanity or abuse. It is a "FEAR" word used liberally to give you low self-esteem and create a narrative to steer you into the "BILLION DOLLAR HEIST". Change the commentary in your head because until you change that commentary, it will be next to impossible for you to create the right environment inside your head, which supports weight loss.

Statements like:

- » **people my age gain weight.**

- » **it's normal in my community.**
- » **I will wear a certain type of clothes, and then it will not show.**
- » **everyone in my family is overweight.**
- » **its all due to my genetics.**

If these statements are running in your head, then these are telltale signs of self-denial. Forget about weight loss if you are using this genre of commentary to not acknowledge your weight gain.

WHY AND HOW DID I GAIN WEIGHT?

Unless you find an answer to these questions, you will not be able to move forward effectively. The answer to why and how will bring you face to face with the choices which have resulted in your weight gain. The choices will point towards the behavioural patterns, which lead you to those choices. The behavioural patterns and preferences will help you single out the beliefs which control the behaviours and choices. Was the weight gain due to:

- » **overeating.**
- » **irregular eating habits.**
- » **too much partying.**
- » **frequent alcohol.**
- » **lack of sleep.**
- » **carb-heavy diet.**
- » **binge eating.**
- » **stress eating.**
- » **any ongoing medications due to some medical**

condition.

It could be anyone or some or all of the above reasons why you gained weight. There has to be a reason for a condition. These are simple and straightforward questions which you have to ask yourself and then address them.

WHY DO I WANT to LOSE WEIGHT?

This is my favourite question which I pose to any prospective client. The answer to this question would decide if I would be ready to take the person onboard my training program. The answer would unravel a lot about the psychological state of the person. If the response was something like: (A)

> » **I want to improve my health.**
> » **I know it can lead to significant health conditions.**
> » **It's detrimental for my families future.**
> » **I want to raise my low self-esteem.**
> » **I want to be happier.**
> » **I want to regain my past weight. I was never like this before.**
> » **I need professional help.**

Responses like these were perfect ground to work on.

But it the responses were on the lines of (B)

> » **I have just got out of a relationship, and I want my ex to feel jealous.**
> » **I want to have a body like that model.**

> » **I want my pictures on Facebook to look hot.**
> » **I want to fit into my teenaged daughter's jeans.**
> » **I am ready to do anything to get rid of this weight.**
> » **I want to do this in the shortest possible time.**
> » **I have tried everything. Let me try you.**

Responses like these would raise red flags for me. I would not sign up people with this genre of reactions. Let me explain why.

The (A) type responses showed that there is a genuine desire to lose weight for self-improvement. There is an acknowledgement that yes, there is a weight issue. The need for weight loss is fuelled by the realisation that this physical state is not an accurate representation of myself. So I have to change it. These type of responses are associated with feelings of being aware, being grounded, realistic, humble and not in search of social validations.

The (B) type responses showed that the desire to lose weight is ego-driven.

The person's life is being impacted by social media in a very major way.

Is not realistic.

Is impatient.

Wants instant gratification.

Is not interested in the process. Only looking at the result.

Could be a status symbol tool.

Considers health a commodity.

You have to analyse your responses here. If most of your answers are the (B) type, let me assure you on one thing. You might be successful in losing weight, but it will never be permanent. You have to first take yourself to type (A) responses if you are really searching for lifelong changes.

My personal experience, if you want to take a note, tells me that the type (B) people are spending way too much time in HIGH BETA brain wave state. A high beta state is associated with feelings of anxiety, stress, jealousy, short temper and inflated ego's. The rate of 80% failure, for me, was because most of my sign-ups were type (B).

NOTE: your responses do not define you as a person. They only tell about your psychological state. You most probably are a fantastic human, regardless of your responses being in type (A) or type (B). But if you want a permanent change, then you have to first bring about the change in your psychology. It is absolutely fine to be wanting a good picture on social media. But that should not be your driving reason for wanting weight loss.

TARGET WEIGHT AND TARGET DATE.

If we embark on a journey, then it's imperative that we know the destination. And if we know the destination, then we should also set arrival date. Your weight loss journey is no different. This is where you need to keep all your preconceived notions about weight loss aside. This is purely science-driven. I am assuming that your responses are type (A) responses.

What you need to understand here is that good weight is a function of :

- **Gender**
- **Age**
- **Height**
- **Blood type**
- **Activity type**
- **Medical history**
- **Body composition**

This is where the "billion-dollar heist" sells you the **"one size fits all"** approach. Beware of that from now.

Ask yourself a few questions like :

- How can the weight loss journey of a teenaged girl be the same as that of a middle-aged woman?
- How can the weight loss of a highly muscular man of 40 years be the same as that of a 40-year-old low muscle man?
- How can the weight loss of 25-year-old young mother be the same as that of a 55-year-old woman who has undergone menopause?
- How can the weight loss of a 45-year-old man be the same as that of a 45-year-old woman?
- How can the weight loss of a 35-year-old female computer operator be the same as that of a 35-year-

old housewife?

So the target weight has to factor in a lot of parameters. A matrix has to be created, and then you arrive at a good weight. Our hormones play a massive role in this. You have to be realistic when you are working out the right weight for yourself.

The most common chart used by the wellness industry is the BMI chart. No doubt it's a useful chart. But it is not the complete picture. What about your BMR?

You will hardly find a mention of this. I find it so funny when you visit a dietician or a weight loss clinic, the first thing done to you is that you are asked to climb on a weighing scale, then your height is measured and then "BANG" your right weight is flashed on to you.

(why would I need to go to a professional for this? BMI charts are available online. Usually weighing scales are available in all households. So I can work out my correct weight by myself. Why should I pay you for this ?)

What you want to get rid of is the excess fat. Not your muscle. Blind weight loss makes you lose fat and muscle. This is where the BMI charts sort of come short. The chart does not factor in your body composition. The chart might show that you are 10 kgs overweight. But you could be a person with a high percentage of muscle weight. So after you factor in that, you could be just 5 kgs overweight.

You could be on some medications due to a health condition. Your weight loss approach will be very different in that case.

You could be of a particular blood type. How does that matter would be your question?

Well, what is blood? It's a chemical.

What is food? It's also a chemical.

So there will be guaranteed food types which will favour certain blood types. How can you ignore that?

One has to be very careful in arriving at target weight. An effort in doing so will go a long way in understanding your own body.

The reason we need to fix a target date is that we want to track our progress. Weight loss is not linear. It's imperative that you know how you are tracking. An open-ended program is not good for weight loss. This is where a realistic approach is so important. A weight loss of 6 to 10 kgs in 3 months is very realistic and achievable. 10 kgs in a month will happen only if you are obese like I was. Or you have starved yourself. Starvation will only do one thing you. It will waste your body. Don't ever do it.

What I have noticed is that most women are generally overweight in the 5 kgs to 15 kgs range. Most men fall into the 10 kgs to 25 kgs range. Obviously, this weight didn't climb onto you one fine nite while you were asleep. It's taken a few years of a particular lifestyle to arrive at where it is now. And my friend, reversing this is very much possible. If you are completely honest to yourself and follow the step by step process, which we are discussing right now, you will achieve permanent change.

WHAT'S THE PLAN

We can have great ideas and a narrative around anything. Without a plan, you can be sure of one thing. **You will never achieve what you have set out for**. (I will discount divine intervention here).

And a plan should be completely objective. It should be based on hard facts and with various scenarios factored in. Let me give you an example.

Consider two men of the same age, height, weight, blood group and body composition. (it can't be more straightforward than this). They sit exactly in the same weight loss matrix. Let's assume they are both 10 kgs overweight. There is only one difference between the two. One has a desk job. The other has a job where he is required to travel anything between 8 to 12 days in a month. This difference has to be factored in. It is vital.

> » THEIR PROGRAMS WILL BE RADICALLY DIFFERENT.
> » THEIR TARGET DATES WILL BE TOTALLY DIFFERENT.

Any good plan or intervention has to factor in all such conditions. A hastily put plan will not take you anywhere.

We have to now put in place a routine which is geared towards :

1. **The psychological aspects. We have to change the core where those beliefs are housed.**
2. **The physical aspects which consist of a balanced diet and routines around it.**

THE PSYCHOLOGICAL PLAN

The psychological plan will be based on carefully observing your behaviour. It might look something like this:

The time I wake up.

Time I sleep.

How much time do I spend on social media?

What type of content do I generally follow?

How much television do I watch?

What's my final activity before sleeping.

What am I doing while I consume my food?

What food do I crave for and when?

What's the time gap between my dinner and sleep time.

How often do I skip my meals?

What is the genre of conversation, when at home and at work, about food?

Do I engage in my hobbies?

What is my relaxation routine?

Do I purchase my groceries?

Do I read labels when I purchase a food item?

Do I supervise or participate in cooking at home (if it's being cooked by someone else)?

How much time do I take to finish a meal?

Do I observe the food that I am consuming?

Do I experiment with different food types?

Do I remember the dreams on waking up in the morning?

What's the first thing I do on waking up.

What's my routine in the first one hour of waking up.

What are my energy levels when I wake up? Am I rejuvenated or tired?

How much do I think about food during the day?

Have you come across a psychological plan on weight loss before this?

Most likely not.

99.9999% plans for weight loss are about calories, fat, alcohol, junk food, fried food, carbs and proteins. Absolutely fine. I don't have an issue on this. But someone, please explain to me just one thing. **Why do they fail?**

Only because they are not addressing the core of the issue, and that core is the belief systems.

There are 24 points listed in the psychological plan. It will be worthwhile if you tick off the ones you definitely do or know about.

I have yet to come across a person who has got all 24 ticked. The maximum a client has ticked was 16. The maximum number of people sit within a range of 5 to 12. How do I analyse this:

0 to 5: will need a lot of help and guidance. The period will be in excess of 6 months.

6 to 9: will need substantial guidance. The period will be about 4 to 6 months.

10 to 14: will need some guidance. The period will be for three months.

15 to 18: requires fine-tuning. The period will be 1 to 3 months.

19 to 21: just requires some helpful directions. No program required.

22 to 24: why do you need me to mate.

Let me translate the above numbers for you. This will help you to get an idea about your psychological state.

(Keep in my mind that we are discussing weight loss here. All these numbers are my own tools which I use when people need help in weight loss. A low number or a high number is just a ready tool. Nothing more).

What your score will tell, is the level your own awareness about yourself. We lead our lives in an unconscious state for the most part of it. We base our understanding of the world around us on a minuscule amount of information coming towards us. Our senses, namely sight, sound, taste, feel and smell, are geared to receive a fraction of the total inputs coming our way. (let me throw in some scientific information here)

The visible spectrum, for instance, is 0.0035% of the entire electromagnetic spectrum. This is a minuscule fraction of the total spectrum visible to human eyes.

The human audible frequency range is from 20 HZ to 20000 HZ. Most animals have a broader range than this.

Our senses have a limited range of operation, and they are all geared towards the external environment. And we end up banking our total reality on this fraction of the actual reality. To add insult to injury, we move about with extremely low levels of awareness. The result is we operate in an even smaller part of the reality.

If you had observed the 24 questions closely, most of the items are around your sleep. (Reread them. It will help)

I jumbled them up on purpose. I didn't want you to catch the pattern. Your primary tool to change any underlying belief will happen during the time you sleep. Many other activities will have to happen, but they are just accessories to the main show. The main show is unfolding during your "**sleep time**". Your angels conspire at that time.

- If you are in the habit of dropping off to sleep while surfing the net, then, you are not creating the right conditions to change any belief system. The last thoughts when you dose off are not of the changed behaviour which you want to install. In this case, the last thoughts are all high Beta wave information.

- If you watch television just before sleeping, then again you will carry the thoughts from the program, you were viewing. It's not the thought of a new belief.

- If you are waking up tired, then it is a clear reflection of your brain activity while you were sleeping. A tired brain in the morning means it has operated in higher frequency zones for most of the time. You need to be in the Delta region for about 25% of the time you sleep. This is extremely important for the repair of your entire body. Poor sleep quality is directly linked with weight gain.

- Going to sleep immediately after your dinner will result in poor sleep quality. Your brain has to remain in a very active state for long periods to digest the food you eat. It will spend more time in higher frequency states.

- If you sleep with thoughts of anger, stress, jealousy, lack, competition or any similar thoughts, you will be reinforcing the belief system, which is the root cause of the behaviour. Such thoughts are high-frequency thoughts. Your sleep quality will be poor.

- If you are engaged in social media right till the time you sleep, then your brain will keep working on the same thoughts and images. This is where you lose control over your brain waves.

- ***** **JUST A REMINDER. THIS IS SCIENCE**** This same science is being used to make you purchase a particular brand, follow a certain celebrity, put you on a path to chase an image, sell products and completely hack your consciousness.**

- It's taken many years for those belief systems to get entrenched in your subconscious. It will take some time and a consistent approach to replace them with different belief systems.

- You very well know what caused your weight gain. It's time you start removing that cause.

- Millions of people lose weight each year. Just a handful can keep it off. Why? The reason is that those handfuls have made a transition at their core. The core is the subconscious.

I am assuming that you are a type (A) person. If not, then I would suggest that you first work towards getting your response to the question," why I want to lose weight", firmly anchored to reasons with a desire for your own betterment. If your intent is driven by ego, media, social pressures, competition or jealousy, then you will find this as a war-like situation. Any ego-driven reason will not be permanent. Media will promote one thing today and a different thing tomorrow and a different thing the day after. A particular model who might be popular today will be replaced by a different face in some time. A diet being a rage today will be replaced by another rage tomorrow. A product which is being hailed as a magic product to-day will be replaced by a bigger magic tomorrow. None of these is permanent except one thing. And that is "YOU".

Let's continue with the plan.

What should be an ideal sleeping routine to harness the brain waves and start implanting the belief systems which support the behaviours we need to achieve a permanent change?

You could be of any ethnicity or nationality or race or colour or size. It doesn't matter at all. You are a human first. The rest are labels for our convenience and creating separation. Every animal sleeps, and so do humans. What I am about to say just now, You most probably will be hearing for the first time. There is a lot of talk about the importance of sleep. It's everywhere. Articles in medical journals. Social media chatter. Talk shows. The statement that I want to make is,

"your sleep is the pivot on which your entire life depends".

You are not to be blamed if you are surprised or sceptical. But the fact remains that the sleeping hours :

- » Cement the belief systems.
- » Sleeping hours clean your brain.
- The human growth hormone which heals your entire body is released only during the sleeping hours.

(Please don't confuse here with the number of hours. It's the quality of the sleep and the routine before and after your sleep).

Meditative practices are anchored in the science of brain waves. A person enters a sleep-like state while being completely awake. The brain waves slow down to low alpha and theta frequency ranges. Accomplished meditators take their brain waves activity down to delta and epsilon ranges. Yogic science has become a rage in the western world. The last two decades have seen an explosion in the interest in these practices. Some estimates put a figure of $1 billion as the size of the business, around yoga, just in the united states. Having been born in India, I used to find the curiosity of Westerners about traditional yogic practices a bit confusing as a child. Yoga was just some obsolete tradition in which people made funny poses. This was in the 60's, 70's and 80's. Something unrelated to all of this but extremely important started unfolding in the 90's. It was information technology. Prior to this, the entire world was only loosely connected in terms of information flow. An event in New York would be known in Delhi after a few days of its occurrence. The commentary was always in the past. This changed drastically in the 90's. The commentary became live. I remember the excitement I had as a young teenager in 1983 when India reached the finals of the cricket world cup in London. The government of India organised the live telecast of the match. It was like front-page headlines. By the time we reached the 90's, live telecasts had become more of a norm than a novelty. Today we are connected through our mobile handsets with the entire world. With this switch, people got connected with each other like never before. It was in the 90's that some extremely serious research was happening around brain wave states. In particular, were the brain imaging techniques. For the very first time, we could see the brain in action. The brain still remains a very secretive organ to study and understand. But our knowledge about it is far more superior today than what it was just 30 years ago. With this research and the technical support, the western and the eastern communities have come together as far as the meditation is concerned. There was this massive wave of people clamouring to learn meditative practices. Let's not translate this into an interest in eastern based religions. The interest was singularly on the techniques to attain those brain wave states which the scientists had decoded in the labs. Fast forward 20 years into the 2010's, the number of yoga centres in a city like Melbourne mushroomed in every nook and corner of the city. It's not out of place today to find yoga instructors being part of fitness centres. This is how far we have come in a mere 30 years. Meditation has become mainstream. I remember, as children, we would associate yoga with hermits and godmen. Today my next-door housewife is a trained yoga instructor.

Why are we even discussing this? Aren't we supposed to be focussing on weight loss?

Of course, that's the intent. The reason I touched upon a little bit of history is that if you want to bring in a change to some deep-seated beliefs in your subconscious, then you have to start mastering your brain waves. The exponential rise in the interest for meditative practices is for that same purpose…. **Mastering the brain waves.**

What people normally do and what they should ideally do?

Let's list them out:

- sleep at odd random times. This is really bad for your body. Have a fixed time to go to your bed and a set time to wake up.

- Will have a heavy meal for dinner and sleep immediately after that. This has to stop. Your dinner should be the lightest meal of the day, and there should be a good gap of 2 hours between your final meal and sleep. Your brain needs to be relaxed.

- Will be browsing their social media feeds right till the time they can't do it anymore. This is a killer habit. It keeps your brain in higher frequency ranges. Sleep has to be a gentle transition from Beta to Delta and back. A real gentle one. This one behaviour takes the gentleness out of the equation. You should be listening to soothing music, not loud, before sleeping or reading some good content. This will help you get excellent quality sleep.

- Will check their mobile phones every time their sleep is broken. This is a disaster. It's normal for us to wake up a few times during the night. But it takes a few seconds to go back to sleep. That action is happening in the Alpha Theta zones. The act of you checking the mobile projects the phone light into your eyes. Your brain reads this as daytime. It climbs towards the beta zone. Simply stop doing this. There is no way around it.

- Will check their mobile feeds as soon as they get up. Stop this. Your brain waves are still in Alpha state when you wake up. Don't get out of your bed at once. Don't open your eyes at once. You are in a critical state at that time. It is almost a meditative state. If you have followed a good sleeping routine, then you need to match it with a good wake up routine. Try to remember the dreams which came to you. That dream is your subconscious talking to you. There would be some key elements, and some will not make sense. You just have to try to remember them. The contours of your subconscious will change if you put in the intent. So guard any external invasion on those subtle messages which your subconscious is trying to send you.

- Your wake up routine should be as relaxed as possible. This is the time when you remain in Alpha and low Beta states for a considerable amount of time. It's an ideal time for a clear-headed planning of the day and reinforcing supporting beliefs.

My friend, I can go on and on regarding the importance of your sleep and the routine which supports a night of good sleep. I had used my own example while I was in Canberra. Remember I would watch television, consume heavy food, consume alcohol and then just drop on my bed. Doing this, I would wake up feeling tired and exhausted. There was no freshness in my body or brain. It was not a good way to start the day. I gained a lot of weight with this routine. And I lost a lot of weight when I changed this routine. And the best thing is I have maintained my weight following a good sleep routine. I clearly remember the phase I was struggling with my weight, and I would sleep with a bagful of toxic thoughts and wake up with a toxic feeling. I would nurture and amplify the same toxicity throughout the day, and the cycle continued. A unique thing about toxic thoughts is that it appears absolutely logical, genuine and caring. We rehearse them so many times that they look harmless and normal within a short while. The best time to break that routine is the sleeping routine. The daily routine is execution time and supporting the positivity. Most of my workshops and lectures have a separate module just on the importance of sleep. Just remember that as a child, you were told a lot of bedtime stories. That child is still inside your subconscious. You are called an adult because of your chronological age and the size of your body. But the programming happened when you were a child. Its time you understand that the **child inside your subconscious** still listens to bedtime stories. Inadvertently you have outsourced that task to television and social media. They don't tell stories. **The ANGELS have been replaced with DEMONS.** It's not good for that child. Take the control back. It's your child. It's your life. It's you.

Ever since I altered the strategy for my clients, the results became very different. The psychology around weight loss is non-negotiable. Sleep is a focus area. Sleep routine has to be journaled. What people notice is that they start finding it much easier to spot the behaviours and choices which are detrimental to their health. And then it starts becoming logical for them to replace those choices.

Take my case. I told you the frequency of my alcohol consumption in that phase. DAILY. I still consume alcohol. But what's the frequency? Maybe half a dozen times in a year. So it has dropped from 365 times to about six times.

And I did not struggle to do that; once I had worked on my core. Prior to that, it was a fight, and I would conclude that I have very low will power—a self-defeating thought. In fact, the period I was with Seb and even after that, I had not touched alcohol. It was natural and without a struggle. We can extend the same logic to our behaviours of food choices and social media addiction. Identify the triggers which lead you to those choices. My trigger to alcohol was the isolation which I had created for myself.

So when do I consume alcohol now?

Not to cover any isolation but to celebrate some special occasion with friends or family.

Food is the biggest reason for our weight gain (at least we think like that). People who are overweight or obese, just like I was, think about food a lot. Their thoughts would be on the next meal while they would have the present one. Quantity is important for them. They eat very fast. They will be doing some activity like watching television, or speaking to someone on their phones or browsing social media or answering an email. For some, it's like a gastronomical event. For some, it is an orgasmic sensation for some an escape from their routine for a little while.

Let me state something unequivocally.

"You have to change the definition of food in your core if you want to lose weight".

As I mentioned in the first part of our conversation, for me, once I had embarked on this transformational journey food was primarily the fuel for my body. This got evolved further. I understood that anything I eat or drink gets converted into me. If I eat junk, it becomes me. If I eat good food, it becomes me. So in a way, the food on the plate was the raw version of me. There was a profound learning for me in this. The learning is that when I look at food it is just not food. It is "ME". The same food gets converted into my cells, my organs, my blood, my hormones, my brain, my muscles, my bones, my DNA, my hair, my nails. Everything that I define as "ME". So if I choose to eat a burger with a fizzy drink and fries, it still gets converted into a "ME". I will become what I put inside my body. **I can't hope to have a good physical aspect of myself by consuming junk and toxic food.**

This changed my relationship with food. I became extremely cognizant of what I ate. I can state with complete confidence and responsibility that this was the result of a new belief system. There is no struggle in making a choice. Its automatically linked with behaviour. That behaviour is emanating from a belief system. The belief system is embedded in my subconscious. This transformation was not overnight with me. It took a while. It has been the same case with most of my clients. Once they developed new belief systems, their healths have been transformed.

We live in a world which is fantastically interconnected thanks to the advancements In telecommunications and transportation. What used to be a luxury just about 50 years ago is now a basic need. The flow of information is seamless. An event occurring in London will be known to everyone within a short time of its occurrence. There is no time gap in information flow. We have to make a choice for ourselves about what information are we chasing and what data are we going to consume. Just as food makes your physical body, thoughts make your consciousness.

Buddha famously said,

"YOU BECOME WHAT YOU THINK".

It was not a slogan. It was a profound scientific fact. You can choose to ignore this or become aware of your thoughts. Because regardless of your choice, there is a multi-billion dollar industry out there which has fully incorporated and embraced this knowledge to harness your fears and vulnerabilities. The corporates are investing billions of dollars in research in mastering your brain waves. They are all trying to plant thoughts inside you. Remember one thing very clearly you are just a number for them. Your favourite celebrity would be getting paid astronomical sums of money for a single Instagram post just for the purpose to grab your attention. Artificial intelligence within the search engines keeps tracking your browsing patterns and history. It works out your preferences and starts feeding you with content matching those preferences. Have you noticed that if you have browsed for some product, let's say a hair product, all the subsequent feeds on your social media account get heavily loaded with similar products? It is not a coincidence. There are serious work and money going on behind the touch screens of your mobile devices. It's the business of brain hacking. It is for you to decide as to whom you will allow hacking your brain. The choice is between the external world and yourself.

I am hopeful that you will be able to start working on the psychological part of your health plan. A physical plan without a psychological plan is an incomplete and non-functional plan. Imagine a friend presents you with the body of a sports car without its engine. This is precisely how a health plan will look like if it has not factored in the psychological part. There are so many diets going around the world—**Keto, G.M., Atkins, Water diet, intermittent fasting, Vegan, Paleo, etc., etc.**

Probably all are good. Probably all give some results.

Then why have they failed in ridding the world of the problem of obesity????

If finding a solution to obesity is so central in reducing life-threatening conditions, then why aren't these diets made central to government health programs and made mandatory for societies to incorporate and follow ????

The reason is implicit. Everyone involved in that industry knows that each of these fads has a shelf life. The shelf life is decided by the amount of noise that can be created around the fad and for how long the noise can be sustained. It's a well-oiled machine. Television channels, famous anchors, celebrities, magazines, advertising agencies, PR agencies, fashion labels, cosmetic industry… you name it. Everyone gets involved. It's not a random approach. It's a plan. They will hack your consciousness and milk a fad at your cost.

Remember how I used to constantly go through content during the phase when I was trying to lose weight. My entire psychology was being governed by a single-minded goal of losing weight. I used to sleep with thoughts of ways to improve my health. Gradually these thoughts were able to change the beliefs in my subconscious, and it has remained like that ever since.

Now that you have understood all of this, my hope is that you will be more observant and not get sucked into it.

THE PHYSICAL PLAN

We have almost reached the end of our conversation. The **weight loss** starts in your head and shows on your body. Just as the **weight gain** starts in your head and appears on your body. I have made an attempt to show you the mind-body link. I will now share with you a very straight forward approach. This same approached helped me lose close to 36 kgs weight from my body (and a few tonnes from my head). Once you have followed the approach and reached this point, you would have found out by now how much weight loss you are targeting.

The physical plan has the following steps:
- Find out your BMI and BMR. Just BMI will not help.
- You must know your blood group.
- Make a diet chart to create a calorie deficiency.

- Make a physical routine to raise your BMR.
- Calculate the percentage of carbs, fats and proteins in your current diet.
- Note down the volume of water you usually consume.
- Note down your current diet over a period of 1 week.

This should suffice as a starting point for you. You need to be as detailed as possible while making notes. These are not for public consumption. Each small notation will act a brick for a solid plan. So be very honest and critical. You will be surprised at what all you eat once you start making notes.

Let's assume here for convenience sake that you are targeting a 10 kgs weight loss. Let's translate this into numbers.

10 kg weight = 80000 kcal approximately.

So you have to make a calorie deficit of 80000 kcal to lose that weight.

Let's assume that your BMR (Basal metabolic rate) is 1900. You can get this number from a good gym or health clinic. This number is critical. This number tells you exactly the number of calories your body burns for its normal daily operations.

You will gain weight when :

Calories consumed > BMR

You will lose weight when:

Calories consumed < BMR

Without this number trying for weight loss is like blindfolding yourself and catching any random bus hoping it was the right one.

If you have made notes of your present diet. The hallmarks of a well-balanced diet are something like this:

* **high protein, low carb, moderate-fat diet.**

* **good portion of the food should be raw or uncooked.**

- **Nuts and seeds an essential component.**
- **Natural unrefined cooking mediums.**
- **No preservatives in ingredients.**
- **Plain drinking water.**
- **Variety.**
- **Colourful.**

Any weight loss regime has a few stages and steps. You might choose to follow any diet subsequently, but the stages are universal. They are:

- **Detox**
- **Executing a weight loss plan**
- **Monitor**
- **Maintenance**

If I was asked to choose the most important part of my weight loss regime, then it will be DETOX. The glaring mistake which I find in the various weight loss programs is the absence of a detox phase. Innumerable clients have shared with me the weight loss programs they were put on by trained dieticians and nutrition experts. Most of those plans did not even find a mention of detox. **Your weight loss will be a non-starter without the detox phase**.

Why is it so?

Your body accumulates a lot of toxins. It could be excess fats, water, sugars, faeces. All of these are contributing to weight gain—the entire body functions as a complex industrial plant. The two primary organs having the task of clearing our body of solid waste are the liver and colon. It is an outstanding practice of cleaning these organs at the start of a weight loss program. There are so many good detox regimes available on the net. Just pick any home-based one. But do it. You will be amazed at what all your body expels once you do this. I have seen people lose 5 to 10 kgs within a span of a week. And all that they loose was solidified faeces in their colons and lots of water. Once your liver and colon are detoxed, your body is in perfect condition to go into a clean diet and hit the start button.

"There is a trick here." Let me share with you.

Due to our toxic diets, our bodies hold a lot of excess water. This water is held primarily due to excess refined sugars that we consume. Remember how I would feast on muffins, cookies, ice creams etc. All the excess sugar molecules in my body were binding with water. As a rough estimate, one sugar molecule binds with four water molecules.

THE FIRST 3 WEEKS OF YOUR WEIGHT LOSS REGIME ARE THE GOLDEN PERIOD.

You can lose a lot of weight if you understand this science and follow your program pedantically.

((((I am assuming you are the type (A) and if you are not then you are working towards becoming one))).

I lost the maximum weight in the first month of my training with Seb. It was such a satisfying and inspiring experience. Seb had clearly explained to me the graph, and I really wanted to get the maximum out of this "GOLDEN PERIOD ". So don't miss this.

Your body gets confused at the start of a new diet.

First, get it detoxed and then commence this new diet. By the time your body works out a new strategy to resist this new diet and regime, its already a few weeks and you have hit the jackpot.

We had assumed a weight loss of 10 kgs for explanation purposes. My estimate in this is that a person targeting a 10 kg weight loss will shed 4 to 6 kgs in the first four weeks. This estimate is based on my personal experience and observations made during the weight loss experienced by my clients.

***** BUT THIS IS THE DANGER ZONE *****

People get overconfident here. They think that this was a cakewalk. They are just looking at the scales and not what their bodies might have expelled to register that weight loss. This is where the psychology of weight loss kicks in. And this is where 90% of people start failing. They ignore the science behind weight loss. A common thought which comes to most people is. **"this is so easy. I can do this anytime."**

Yes, it is easy provided you have registered the science.

No, it's not permanent because you have not grasped the psychology.

That's why you hear this statement so often, **"I lose some weight so easily, and then it all comes back within no time."**

Is it making sense to you now? I hope it is.

That 4 to 6 kg weight loss in the first four weeks would mainly consist of water loss. The actual **"FAT LOSS"** might be 1 kg or 1.5 kgs.

Nevertheless, its a weight loss and we have to utilise this window. Once your body has lost all this water and some fat, it gets steady from here. Say you register 4 kgs weight loss in the first four weeks. A reasonable expectation would be to have a steady weight loss of about half a kg per week from here on. Anything more is a bonus.

Like in my case, I went over and above with my suggested routine, and the results were in line with the effort. Plus I was carrying a lot of excess weight to start with. The most crucial thing in this entire journey is that "YOU HAVE TO ENJOY IT ". That will happen only if there are some fundamental changes in your core beliefs. Else it remains a task which you are forced to perform. This is the psychology I am alluding to again and again. If you consider this as a task, then it will feel like a task. You will not enjoy the food you consume as your thoughts would keep going back to your old diets. The routine will appear to be a prison sentence. There will be a feeling of lack inside you. The mind will translate the routine as a means to exclude you from the "good times ".

And that enjoyment can happen if there is a fundamental change in your core beliefs. That's why I am emphasising so vehemently on the psychological aspect of weight loss.

Coming back to the present scenario. Let me share a few more simple tricks which will help you lose that 10 kg weight. And these are time tested and scientifically backed techniques. They have been present all the time, but their importance and explanations are not amplified because these are to be kept "SECRET ".

(1) CHEW YOUR FOOD WELL.

You must have heard this as a side talk only. Never as a main discussion point. Weight gain is aided in a big way by overeating. People who are overweight generally eat extremely fast. I used to do that. They have this psychological bonding with food. Eating **food fast is a disaster**. There is a hormone called *ghrelin* in your stomach, which acts as a messenger between your brain and stomach to register that you are full. It takes about 20 minutes for this circuit to complete. And by that time we could have eaten twice or thrice more than what we should. There is a lot of science around the trigger mechanism of these hormones. It will be an interesting read for you. So this particular overeating habit can be curtailed by the single act of chewing your food really well.

It's just not a simple time delay tactic. It has fantastic benefits. More than 50% of the process of digestion of the food we eat has to happen in our mouths. We as humans have a digestive system which performs the best when it receives the food in a semi-liquid state in our stomach. Proper mastication of the food breaks it down to a state where it is best digested. The micronutrients get released and are absorbed by our digestive tracts. Chewing the food well reduces the stress on the oesophagus. The food in a semi-liquid state will help in eliminating conditions like acidity, bloating and constipation. Plus it will help you know in good time that you are full now.

I will give you my example here. The moment I understood this simple thing and started following it, my food consumption went down to half. That's a lot of extra food I was eating. So incorporate this "SECRET "act.

(2) DON'T DRINK ANY WATER WHILE EATING.

This is another major habit which makes us overeat. The masticated food has to spend some time in your stomach and upper gut region to be properly digested. If you drink water or any beverage while you are eating, the undigested food travels much faster out of the stomach. The feeling of fullness will be delayed because the hormone will not get triggered.

(3) DON'T WATCH TELEVISION OR YOUR SOCIAL MEDIA FEEDS.

I simply can't emphasise enough on this one aspect. Your undivided attention has to be on that one activity of eating. Television simply takes that attention away from food. You end up not chewing the food well. You end up eating more than your hunger. And the worst is that you have not enjoyed the food.

(4) NO WATER FOR AT LEAST 30 MINUTES AFTER YOUR MEAL.

For the same reason as above that you need the food to remain in your guts for that time for it to be processed properly. Lots of people have the habit of drinking water immediately after finishing their meals. If you have chewed your meal well and spent a good time finishing it, then there will also not be any requirement of water to push down the food stuck in our oesophagus. The term to be remembered here is "**MINDFUL EATING** ". I used to require drinking water so many times while having my meal only because I would be eating real fast and big chunks of food would get stuck in my oesophagus. To push them down, I would need water. So stop doing that.

(5) NEVER DRINK COLD WATER.

There is enough scientific evidence around this simple-looking aspect. I will just limit our conversation around weight loss. Drinking cold water reduces the temperature of our body. So the body has to work to bring it back to the average level, which is about 98.6 degrees Fahrenheit. The stomach walls shrink when you drink cold water. Male adults need about 3.7 litres and female adults about 2.7 litres on a daily basis. Coldwater reduces that thirst. I will be so pleasantly surprised if you are consuming these recommended quantities of water. A reduced intake of water has severe long term effects on our health. One of them is that we misinterpret a "THIRST SIGNAL WITH A HUNGER SIGNAL". This is a rampant habit with all overweight people. A lot of our thirst is replaced with food. We don't realise that our body is 72% water—lack of water results in dehydration. Overweight, people generally have dry and lifeless skin.

(6) CHANGE THE COMPOSITION OF YOUR FOOD INTAKE.

I can confidently state that this bit of information or secret is the "**MOTHER OF ALL BATTLES WITH THE BULGE** ". Our typical food composition is carbohydrate loaded. A look at any meal intake routine will be something like 70% to 80% carbs. The remainder will be proteins and fats. **THIS IS A DISASTER**. Simply understanding this one single aspect of your chemistry will put you on a path of good health forever. We should be getting at the most 60% of our calorie requirements from carbs for a healthy adult of optimum weight. (*kindly refer to an excellent medical site to match up your carb requirement based on gender, age, optimum mass and height*). Anything more will get stored as fat. So if you are trying to lose weight, then a very effective way is to reduce your carb intake to about 25% and increase the protein intake. This has immense health benefits other than just weight loss. Overweight people generally suffer from diabetes, hypertension and cholesterol issues. A high protein low carb diet helps them a lot in reducing and reversing those conditions.

There is enough **medical research and explanations** regarding all the six, so-called "**SECRETS** ", I just revealed to you. Read that type of content. It doesn't cost a cent, and it's priceless. You don't need to do a PhD to know about such facts. And neither do you need permission from state authorities to access such information. It's not classified. But it certainly requires one thing, and that is "you want "to gain knowledge. Only then will you be able to answer your "**WHY'S AND HOW'S** ".

Any person who has come in my contact for weight loss has been taken through this process. It's indeed a very satisfying feeling when you become part of those happy journeys. I don't recommend crash diets or gruelling gym routines to anyone. The best form of exercise is a brisk walk around the block you live in. 4 to 6 walks a week are the best. I personally prefer walks now. There is a healthy mix of weight training sessions in my routine. But not the type I executed during my stint with Seb.

My conversations with my clients are around fresh vegetables, nutrition through nuts and seeds, suitable cooking mediums, salad recipes, any new content about food and so on. Putting a robust and dynamic program in place is non-negotiable. It's best to break down the weight loss into chunks. A 10 kg weight loss will happen in a period of 60 to 90 days, provided the plan is followed.

You now have a complete blueprint of an approach which addresses the psychological and physiological aspects of a weight loss journey. I have shared my personal and professional experiences with you. This is not the holy grail of weight loss. But yes, it is indeed an approach which has seen a lot of success. I encourage you to follow the road map we have discussed.

If you want to just cherry-pick some part of the map, it's okay. You can always come back to the complete plan in case you feel lost. You have it with you from now.

Simple maps are the best maps.

The more significant part of the wellness industry is geared towards presenting a strategy which needs to appear **sophisticated, elusive, exotic, magical, instantly gratifying, fashionable and celebrity-driven**. Do you have to ask your self one simple question? Am I looking for a permanent change, or do I just want to be part of a blind crowd, following a fad? This one answer will decide the route you choose.

The time we have spent in this conversation until now will never come again. It's history. But the information you now have has the potential to change anything in your life. The information is based on my personal life experience. I know how it felt to be fat. I have experienced first hand the frustrations of failing to lose weight. My body knows what craving is. I know how it feels to be led into believing that weight loss is a straight-line approach. I have made a humble attempt at sharing those experiences and more with you. I conduct regular workshops for trainers as well. These workshops are not about workouts and diets. I am very well aware that the participants know much more than me on those aspects. These workshops are towards the "mind "part. Our knowledge is useless if it cannot be transferred to a recipient. Communication skills, emotional quotients, flow states etc. is what these workshops are based on. I keep doing my part in this quest of equipping people with tools for self-transformation.

Maintenance

An essential part of a weight-loss regime is the maintenance part. Once you reach your target weight, then you need to put in a regime in place which keeps the weighing scales in your desired range. For this to happen, the most important aspect is to be extremely vigilant of your behaviours. It's easy to slip back to your old ways. One cheat meal becomes two meals within no time. Be true to yourself. If you have been able to make a change in your core, then it's impossible to shift back to your old ways. Your new way of life should become permanent. It should not be a task. Maintain a diary. Work on the calorie bank concept. It works. Try it and be amazed at the results.

"When the individual has balanced the world of the consciousness with that of the physical senses will he experience reality in
a purer form. When a person flows from the centre; a place where
all the earth and stars are contained, then we find balance and
happiness"

BHAGAVAD GITA.

"When you feel the suffering of every living thing in your heart,
that is consciousness"

BHAGAVAD GITA

CHAPTER NINE

SEEKING SOME HELP FROM A LITTLE BUDDHA

I can draw a line between two stages of my life.

On one side is a man who thought that he had complete control over his life. Every event was a win or a loss. He knew the most. He knew the best. He could never be at fault. A difference of opinion implied personal insult or betrayal. Consumption was the purpose of life. Social validation the benchmark of success. A man who considered anger as a tool to subjugate. Raised voice as a sign of masculinity.

On the other side of that line is Me. I make it a point to meet the man on the other side each day of my life. He needs healing. He needs to be heard. I know that I need to be patient with him. I have been able to make him understand a few things. A few are still pending. There are so many facets of life which I still don't understand. So whenever that man poses those questions, I ask for his patience. Together we seem to be on a journey where both of us are helping each other to erase that line which divides us. The line which separates us. We both know that a day will come when that divide is removed forever. A day will come when only a Me will remain. **A new me.**

I am not engaging in a cinematic dialogue over here. This sort of conversation happens within all of us at all times. It's some kind of a constant struggle to be something more than what we are today. There is something inside us which seems to ask for something else. We think it's asking for more. There appears to be a breakdown of communication between that voice and us. It's that small soft voice which gets drowned in the cacophony of our everyday routines. We don't register that a thick wall of separation gets erected between that voice and us. Life has become like a maddening race to an imaginary finish line. This appears to be a cliché, but there is no other way to describe it. I am not in any way suggesting you to become a hermit. Not at all. I am alluding to the race within our consciousness. For a person who lives in rented accommodation, his benchmark of success will be to become the owner of a small apartment. He feels satisfied when he achieves that. But almost immediately, he starts planning for a bigger apartment. That becomes his new goal. If he is not able to accomplish that goal, he becomes a failure within himself. If he succeeds in getting to that goal, he sets the next target of a bigger one or a target of a second apartment. And this chain of events repeats with every aspect of his life. It happens with each one of us. Most of our frustrations are due to our failure to reach the finishing line of that imaginary race. And mind it, we run several races simultaneously. That's why the word milestone is used so generously in any commentary around the topic of progress. The only measure of our progress is a number.

We have been made to believe that we are numbers.

How much you earn? A number.

How many houses do you own? A number.

What's your bank balance? A number.

How many cars you have? A number.

How many holidays do you take? A number.

Where do you live? An implicit number linked to your affordability.

Which restaurant do you dine at? An inherent number related to your status.

It's sort of fashionable to post quotes of Christ, Buddha, Rumi, Mother Teresa or Swami Vivekananda on our social media feeds. It gives us a mask to wear.

Does it matter how many houses Christ owned or not?

Does it matter how many dresses Mother Teresa had or not?

We want to fool ourselves into believing that these are our ideals. We use their names and images to create a narrative about ourselves to hack into the consciousness of the society we move about. Had there been an iota of truth in that belief, then your behaviours in daily life would have been very different. I have observed, with unfailing consistency, conversations about Buddha or Nelson Mandela being peppered with gossip about some person who was having an affair with a colleague. I have just picked up one example. It seems that scandal is the common ground where we bond with each other. Being judgemental about everyone has become our birthright. We create a bubble of illusion around our consciousness by using words as positivity, gratitude, empathy, kindness and acceptance. It feels good to us, and it feels useful to people around us. But that bubble bursts at the first traffic signal when the driver of the vehicle in front of us delays moving for a few seconds. Out comes the anger, impatience, judgements, raised voices, throwing of hands in the air with disgust and maybe some adjectives. The Buddha, the Nelson Mandela, the Mother Teresa don't exist for us at that moment. Their message, which we conveniently use as slogans to augment the narrative of ourselves, has not gone into our core. A small prick in the form of an event can burst that bubble. Our real core comes out like a hissing cobra from it's burrow. The game repeats in various ways throughout our daily routines. We hardly notice it. Blissfully ensconced inside the illusion of our bubble we keep trudging the journey of our lives unconsciously.

Numbers are significant for us. The mention of a name like Buddha or Christ brings out an image of billions of followers. Using those names is most likely an attempt by our ego to usher some of those followers on to following us. The crafty business person inside us uses these names and symbols to hack into the consciousness of our audience. The commentary inside us is firmly anchored to the belief of external validation. I will use these quotes so that the world knows I follow Buddha. I will help a poor and ensure that the world knows and acknowledge how generous I am. I will post patriotic jingoism on my social media handles so that the world knows about my allegiance. It's all geared towards numbers and social validations.

It's high time we ask ourselves a few blunt questions. Will, I end up being any less a Buddha if I help a single poor with the genuine desire to help him? Will I be any less a Christ if I extend my hand forward to extricate someone from a personal issue?

And more important than the above questions, Does social validation matter if I have genuinely imbibed the message of a Christ or a Buddha?

The dividing line I mentioned about myself was drawn around the year 2017. I will not absolve myself and sit on a high horse trying to preach righteousness to you. A part of me still meanders to the other side of that line. But I have become very metacognitive now, which means that I observe my thoughts at all times. It's not easy for me to get sucked into a conversation unconsciously. This single act of observing my thoughts keeps me firmly anchored to my core. If I have food, then all my attention is on the food. If I am having a conversation, then my entire focus is on that conversation. There is no desire to prove my point to anyone. I know that there is something unimaginably massive of which we all are a part of. That enormous thing communicates with us through that small soft voice. We can hear that voice only if we demolish that wall of separation we have created. I have had fleeting moments of that experience. Just fleeting. Nothing more than that. I have experienced that voice whenever I have tried to help anyone without an agenda, without expectation of a return favour and without seeking any social validation. It's not essentially about monetary help. Sometimes just a gentle help to someone dealing with emotional trauma or someone looking for an objective non-judgemental analysis of a situation. Each of such events brings out a little bit of the Buddha or Christ from inside my core.

That fleeting connect has been enough to change my internal chemistry. Those moments were successful in bringing down the walls of separation. I lose the sense of time, hunger, sleep, fatigue, pain and self in those fleeting moments. There is a scientific name for that state. Its call a Flow state. The bulk of my current work is around such states and how to achieve them.

It is with utmost awe when we speak about entrepreneurs like Jeff Bezos, Bill Gates or Warren Buffett. They are first-generation entrepreneurs who have rewritten the rules of wealth creation. What they have created in the last 30 years simply puts to shame what some of the largest business conglomerates did in 150 years. Same is the case when you speak about adventure sports, traditional sports, arts, music and fine arts. Now and then, a Maverick comes out and rewrites the rules. And this has become a more regular feature since the late 1990s.

I used to be fascinated by just reading about the exploits of these people. Nothing more. I always thought that they were more gifted and had very high levels of motivation and will power. These were convenient explanations until I saw an interesting article about happiness during my net surfing sessions when I had shifted to Melbourne. One item led to another till I reached an article on some god forsaken concept of **flow**. The author was **Mihaly Csikszentmihalyi**. I know it's a total tongue twister. And trust me, this gentleman did end up twisting my complete approach towards life. His work on Flow states is of epic proportions when it comes to ultimate human performance and peak states. His works have led me to develop a deep interest in the concepts of human consciousness. That interest, combined with pieces of training on spiritual practices in India has removed layers and layers of mist from my understandings about the way the human mind operates.

When a world record is broken, most observers will see hard work, toil, motivation, training, natural ability and will power. Absolutely yes.

But from where does that level of motivation and will power come?

It comes from flow states.

So when I see a world record being broken, I see a flow state at work. Same was the case when we spoke about people like Jeff Bezos etc. they have mastered flow states. If you and I are at level 1, then these individuals are at level 10. That's 900% more than us. What these people do in one year will take people like you and me ten years. And I am being very modest here.

Flow is a science and it's been embedded in spiritual practices the world over. There has always been a shroud of mystery thrown over this knowledge. But in the last 2 or 3 decades that cover has been pulled away. We are now beginning to understand our hidden powers. My work is totally centred around explaining and training people of that potential. Once you come face to face with that potential, it becomes a matter of choice from there. You can choose to unleash the beast inside you, or you can choose to ignore it and continue with the daily struggles of a mundane life.

You must have observed that there has been a sudden spurt in the usage of terms such as **transcendental meditation, chakra healing, kundalini, 3rd eye activation, Akashi records, quantum reality, tantra, the law of attraction, past life regression, hypnosis, reiki, pranic healing**, etc. All of these and many more are based upon energy systems and brain wave states. The names might sound ancient or spiritual, but these practices are based upon solid scientific concepts. Each one of these is being researched scientifically with verifiable and measurable scientific evidence. It is just a start so as to say. Our understanding of the human mind and body can only grow from here. I personally expect that by the year 2040, a lot of our education systems, medical practises and social engagements will see a significant shift towards energy systems. Most of the concepts of today, which are called cutting edge and state of the art, will look primitive within the next decade. I can see a definite shift towards a raised consciousness. It's still a tiny community, but it is multiplying. And let's not confuse ourselves over here with religion. The debate over which religion is better than the other will keep happening for some more time to come. That debate is alive due to the low level of consciousness of the larger human population. As the percentage of people with higher consciousness grows, a stage will come where these debates will not be part of our societies. Religions will survive, and they will thrive.

It is said that all good things come to an end. We have reached the end of our pleasant conversation. You must have noticed that I have always used the word conversation. For any discussion or dialogue, there should be two people. I still consider myself having a conversation with the author of the book I might be reading. There is an instant connection which I experience. Thanks to the internet, it is incredibly convenient to look up images and videos of the author. This has made my reading habit like a conversation happening in real-time.

So where am I and where are you?

I am embedded in these words as you read them. And you are that voice which is translating these images into words and giving you a meaning. I started this conversation by mentioning that we are all a part of a much larger combined consciousness. An innumerable number of people must have conspired to make this conversation possible.

Siddhartha was a prince, a married man and a father before he raised his consciousness to a level where the entire world calls him Buddha. The rough translation of Buddha is the enlightened one.

Agnes Gonxha Bojaxhiu was an Albanian nurse who worked in the slums of modern-day Kolkata. We know her by the name of Mother Teresa due to her selfless work for easing human pain and suffering.

Mohandas Karamchand Gandhi was a lawyer, a husband, a father. People started calling him as Mahatma Gandhi due to the level of his consciousness and the work he did for humanity.

Our complete history is replete with such names. None of these people was some unique creations. They were just like us to start with. But once they established a connect with that small soft voice inside them, they became what we know then as today. There is an intelligence residing within all of us. I am not speaking about the degrees we get upon completing a coarse or the titles which get bestowed upon us due to those degrees. That is just information. If you have three degrees and I have one, then all this implies is you have more information compared to me on specific subjects. That's all that it means. Buddha did not attend an elite degree college to learn the art of mastering his consciousness. He went inside himself to unearth the knowledge of the entire cosmos residing within himself.

The intelligence, I am referring over here, is the combined consciousness of the whole creation from its inception to eternity.

The names used above is for the purpose of reminding you and me of what we can achieve to serve humanity. That is the prime purpose of the birth of every human. The bridge to that intelligence is only through a raised level of consciousness. Saint Kabir was a 15th-century mystic and a poet with no formal education. Five centuries post his demise there are doctorates being presented to people who spend many years trying to decode and understand his wisdom. The knowledge which he propagated was a result of his connecting to his inner self.

We can choose to remain in the constant rut of an invisible race driven by a low state of consciousness. Or we can raise our awareness to transcend that bridge and have a vision far more significant than what we have now. The science is there, and so is the evidence pointing towards that intelligence. All you need to do is to start talking to that small soft voice. A child studying in year eight is considered having more information than a child studying in year seven. The complete knowledge of those seven years is within the child studying in year eight. His education is built upon the basis of his learnings in the previous years. This is how he keeps going to the next class. Imagine the information and knowledge of 14 billion years of cosmic activity which has produced the creature called human. Yes, that's the knowledge each one of us is holding inside us. And just have a look at what we have got ourselves entangled in?

I have started on a journey to connect with that vast knowledge hidden inside me. As mentioned earlier, I have had fleeting moments of that connect. Even those fleeing moments have changed my internal chemistry. There are no words to describe that state. I am no more concerned with any labels attached to myself. I just know the purpose of my life, and I hope that our conversation helps you to find yours.

CONCLUSION OR A FRESH START?

This work might have my name as the author. But this was not possible without the presence of many people in this journey. A few stand out. I say that because this journey would have been very different if they had not appeared. As I had mentioned at the start of this conversation, this is not a fictional narration. Each and every character is real. I am listing a few of those names here.

Sebastian Jago.

My trainer who resurrected my failing health. He might have worked only on my health but what I learnt from him was much more than just health. His communication skills, his subtle ways of engagement, the care factor and humbleness. Those aspects have got embedded into my core.

Dr Mamta Kapoor.

My close friend who introduced me to the technical concepts of psychology. Her in-depth knowledge about the subject has been of invaluable help to me in formulating the various training modules which I incorporate in my business now. I could not have understood the concepts like the inner child and core, had it not been for her. Her constant encouragement helped me to back myself and embark on a new career.

Pankaj Kapoor.

My childhood school friend who stands like a rock behind me. He was and remains my personal back office. His help in organising my seminars, making all travel reservations, looking after the logistics in the initial part of my business, help during a medical crisis in my family and just being there in my low moments have all played an important role in my journey.

Rakesh Arora.

My school time senior, a friend and my business associate. The trust and faith that he puts in me are very humbling. I feel liberated to experiment and innovate due to his presence in my life. I think and behave like a young boy in his company. His presence is calming and reassuring.

There are numerous people who have helped me on this journey. The list will be very long. They have appeared in my life at various times. They are My Angels. I have this firm belief that there are many more angels who are yet to emerge. The appearance of angels is the direct result of my intent. These words might be coming out of me. But the meanings were created with them. What we call life is just a sequence of many moments strung together. Some moments stand out, but the fact remains that each moment is in place due to the previous moment. About five decades ago, when two young adults must have held me in their arms for the first time, they would not had the slightest of inklings that the baby they were carrying would be an author one day. My story was in the making from that moment. Each one of us has a story in us. I have been able to put it across just due to these angels. They have conspired in making me do this. The moment we start acknowledging the intrinsic relationship we have with the entire cosmos, that very moment we experience the dropping of the various masks which we wear. We think that by adorning these masks, we camouflage our vulnerabilities from the outer world. In actual, these masks are just creating an illusion for ourselves. These masks only create separation. The roadside eatery in Goa, where I used to have a snack, has an equal share of contribution in my journey. Its presence is no less critical than my meeting with the CEO of some large corporations in the plush settings of a five-star hotel. My task is to continually erase that line of separation between that soft small inner voice and my current self. That voice is the bridge to super consciousness. And that superconsciousness is that large data bank of knowledge gained over the last 14 billion years of creation.

I continue to train people on these concepts just as

I keep learning the art of removing that layer of separation between my consciousness and my current reality. Over the last few years, I have made some of the most endearing relationships. It seems as if someone conspired for these relationships to take shape. The only reasoning I could give was the presence of a combined consciousness which brought so many people of the same frequency together. You can call it synchronicity or coincidence, but what I have observed is that these events are occurring at a much higher rate with me now than a few years ago. Help appears in the form of people or events. Just as I am successively dropping the various masks, the invisible race is becoming more apparent. Things which I used to chase a decade ago have lost their allure. I find a book on consciousness much sexier than a branded shirt. Organising free workshops for children are way more rewarding than a paid one for a corporate. I proactively take steps to connect with nature. Because that is what we are—an expression of nature. The workshops which I conduct are mostly experiential now. The venue could be the Himalayas or the beaches of Australia. Doing these workshops in the wilderness brings out a new dimension in learnings. What started as a weight-loss endeavour has morphed into a quest for self-realisation. My journey is not to unravel the origins of the cosmos. My search is just to enable myself to experience the working of the cosmos within myself. At one point, I thought that I had wasted way too much time in my life by not being on this path of self-realisation earlier. But then I understood that it was my ego which was making me draw that conclusion. There is nothing like time. It's a concept to create separation. The past, the present and the future are all happening at this precise moment. I try to explain these concepts in my workshops. All of us chase happiness. Till the time that chase is external, it will never get completed. The moment it becomes internal, the pursuit ceases to be. A pillow fight with my siblings or children is still as much enjoyable as it was five decades ago. A non-sensical talk with a childhood friend always brings out the giggles from grown-up men. The site of the rainbow still brings out a smile of awe. The reason why there are so many unhappy people in the world is that we have made our happiness linked with things.

Happiness is a state of our consciousness. It's internal. Things are external. That's why an expensive car ceases to give joy within a short period of its purchase. It loses allure. We then start chasing something else. Stop this. Just take a short break and observe yourself. What seems elusive to you is sitting within you. This is the reality. You could be a Christian, a Muslim, a Buddhist, a Hindu, an atheist or some cult follower. The fact remains that happiness is internal. Only a raised consciousness will allow you to accept this truth.

There is fantastic content readily available for our consumption on the subjects of consciousness and good health. Technology has presented us with this opportunity to avail. Just imagine if the internet was available to Buddha. An egocentric response to this suggestion would be like; There would be so many more followers of Buddhism. Do you know that there was no image of Buddha for 500 years after his demise? His teachings were relayed from one generation to the next. There was only the image of the bodhi tree, under which Siddhartha became Buddha. His consciousness had transcended to a level where his teachings did not require internet to sustain. He had plugged into the superhighway of information flow, the human heart. He was not seeking external validations. Imagine if you get two simultaneous invitations for dinner with Mother Teresa or the model with the hottest body you have been surfing for. Problem is you can choose only one. Most likely, 99.99999% of humanity will feel blessed to have a meal with the saint of the gutters, Mother Teresa. The meal would be frugal—the setting most basic. But we will feel the presence of divinity if we could have that moment. Our intrinsic nature is to be divine. But we end up drowning that nature with the external noise. Mother Teresa left her body in 1997, and Buddha left his in 483 B.C. you and I will leave ours in the next few decades. The message left by Buddha and Mother Teresa will remain relevant until eternity. We have to think about the message we are creating.

My personal take on this is that the intrinsic motivation of the cosmos is the uplifting of human consciousness. And the cosmos puts its entire weight behind any thought which works in that direction. If a thought is without agenda of seeking benefit for ourselves and is geared for benefiting anything in nature, then it gets help from everywhere. I used to use words like coincidences and synchronicity. Now I feel it's the basic rule of the cosmos to throw all its weight behind any thought which promotes uplifting of human consciousness. This book started with my personal journey of weight loss and has reached its completion with my quest for self-realisation.

I am not a guru or a mystic who has attained enlightenment. I am just a fellow traveller like yourself. The only concept which has got anchored within me is that the cosmos is not operating on coincidences. It is working on an effective plan. And our only means to connect with the cosmos is a thought. Each and every thought will invite a response. It's a colossal energy field which surrounds everything that exists. A planet or a cell are all made up of atoms. An atom is made up of subatomic particles. Those particles are made up of even smaller particles known as the God particles. But what are those God particles made up off? **Just waves of energy**. There is scientific evidence for that. It's undeniable. A thought is just an energy wave. It can be measured. Should we not then conclude that everything is an expression of that energy field. Our realities are our creations. If we become more observant to the events around us and within us, then our interpretations of those events will change. An over-dependence on interpretations from an agenda-driven commentary will create chaos within ourselves. I keep observing my responses to all of these events. It has helped me to experience a peaceful state of mind. Each time I experience any chaos in my mind, the immediate realisation is that there is a part within me which is not accepting that event. There is still some egocentric region which needs healing. My rendezvous with that small soft voice has become more frequent now. What I have observed is that voice becomes more audible when I connect to nature. Walking barefooted on the beach or going for a hike in the forest or swimming in the mighty Ganges provide me with so much pure and unadulterated pleasure.

My favourite workshops are those which I conduct with young children. The inner child comes alive the moment I am surrounded by these young minds. That inner child feels no pressure about being judged while I am in the company of young children. My audience thinks that I am there to teach them something. Yes, I do share some life tools which could be of some help, but the biggest reason for my being there is to experience that innocent energy which these children exude. The inner child within my core finds an instant connect with that energy. And that experience is universal. We simply have to observe it. We could be not liking a particular person due to whatsoever reason. But we find it extremely hard to harbour the same dislike for that person's infant or young child. Our core simply does not have the capacity to harbour those beliefs. We experience the nonexistence of ego at that moment. That's our true self. Non-egoistic and non-egocentric. I have been able to overcome a lot of my negative emotions about a few people just by connecting to my inner child.

We so many times see that children play and often get into small fights. But they are back to playing with each other in no time. Those minor disputes are not nurtured or festered. That's the capacity with which we are born initially. It has a scientific name as well. It's called the re-fractory period. Shorter the period, better is our capacity to overcome feelings of hate, jealousy, anger, disgust and sadness. Why is that as children, we were wired to overcome all such emotions, and as we grew, we lost that capacity. The reason is social conditioning. It was so simple to enjoy our lives as children. There were no biases or judgements in our behaviours. It required an extraordinary effort from someone to make us unhappy. Now we spend most of our time in a state of unhappiness.

I am on this journey to raise my consciousness. I read and follow a few great minds. I encourage you to start making an effort to connect with your small soft voice. There is nothing as late. It's always a start. Let me assure you of one thing. You will never regret connecting with yourself. You are your angel.

My life has become much more straightforward than what it used to be. I have personal responsibilities like all of us. There are challenges around the business, similar to any fledgling venture. The shift in consciousness has altered the processing of these responsibilities and challenges. Preferences have changed. A road trip crisscrossing the farms is far more enjoyable than a short air trip. Having a meaningful conversation with an author is way higher in priority than a movie at the cinem's.

And here I am sipping coffee at the departure terminus of the Melbourne international airport on the 14th of December 2019, waiting to catch my flight to Delhi and giving finishing touches to this beautiful conversation with an unseen expression of myself. Something similar happened in August of 2015. Same airport. Same destination. The only thing different is the not so same me. My physical body is only a cover over a consciousness. That consciousness has evolved during this period of 4 years. I wouldn't want to pass judgement over the trajectory that-my consciousness has taken.

Was it a mere coincidence that this book reached you?

Just keep one fact in your mind before you answer that question. The cosmos doesn't operate on coincidences. The word coincidence is a human creation to mask our limited understanding of the cosmos.

I take leave not from you but,

I take leave from my expression in a form called you.

Till we meet again,

Gratitude.

THESE ARE A FEW OF MY FAVOURITE THINGS...

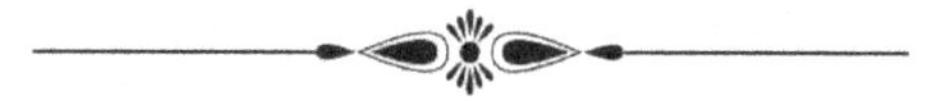

Superfoods: Almonds, Walnuts, Chia Seeds, Flax Seeds, Manuka Honey, Aloe Vera, Indian Gooseberry, Wheatgrass.

Beverage: Black coffee, Lime mint water, Cacao drink.

Cuisine : South Indian, Mediterranean, Anything cooked with love.

Workout: A long brisk walk, Bodyweight exercise, Free water swim.

Hobbies: Writing poetry, Historical reading, Any genre of music.

Unwinding regime: Cooking, Gardening, Connecting with childhood mates.

Hour of work : 4 a.m.

Mode of transport: Drive, Driven, Rail, Cruise, Air. (in the order as mentioned)

City: Melbourne, Goa, London, Bangalore, Istanbul, Cairns. (in the order as mentioned)

Movie: Finding Nemo(my daughter made me watch it at least a thousand times)

Speaker: Osho, Dr Dispenza, Bill Clinton.

Author: Too many to chose from.

Quote: 'You become what you think by Buddha.'

Outfit: Worn out shorts and a T.

Coach: Sebastian Jago, Dr Mamta Kapoor.

Season: Winters.

Aroma: The smell of earth after the first rain.

Sound: the sound of waterdrops falling slowly from a leaking tap into a half-filled bucket.

Animal: Stray dogs.

Movie: Les Miserables (1957)

Actor: Guru Dutt

Actress: Madhubala

Poet: Saint Kabir

Singer: STING

Musical band: ACDC

A FEW THINGS I AVOID COMPLETELY...

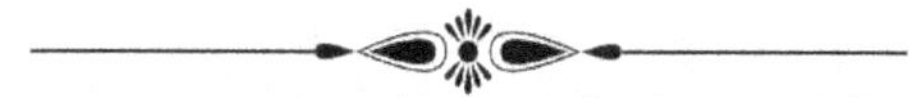

Gossip of any shape and size.

Late nights unless travelling or some extremely important celebration.

Late dinner.

Speaking out of turn.

Speaking unnecessarily.

Religion.

Being loud.

Cuss words.

Expensive clothes. (I prefer discounted clothes)

Specialists of any field. (I prefer amateurs or startups)

Business-class air travel. (unless being upgraded)

Fancy restaurants. (I prefer local and lively places)

Lunch or dinner meetings.

Chemical sprays of any type. (body deodorant has to be natural, room freshener has to be natural, the surface cleaner has to be natural)

No television. (exception is live cricket or Australian open)

Never check my social media feed till about 8 a.m.

No social media engagement from half an hour before sleeping.

Never charge any school for training.

Use of complicated terms in my lectures. (people switch off)

Posting of personal content on social media. (don't seek social validation)

WHAT DO I LOOK FORWARD TO?

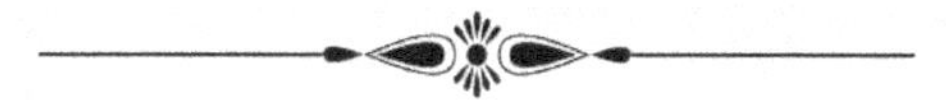

As a world citizen:

A complete overhaul of the education systems around the world wherein health becomes the fulcrum on which an individual is developed.

Children till the age of 10 years are taught concepts of hygiene, farming, punctuality, art forms and local languages mainly in an experiential format. They should be encouraged to play as much as possible and express themselves. There should be no examinations based on academic subjects for these children.

The defence and education budgets of the country should be the same.

Health should be exclusive with the state.

Junk food should be taxed in the same way as tobacco and alcohol.

As a professional:

I would want to train myself further on nutrition and the mind concept. The content emanating from my platforms has to be continually simplified and localised. The platform should attract talent wanting to express itself and enrich the experience of people who come onto the platform. It should act as a bridge between science and spirituality.

Personally:

Maintain a healthy body. My yardstick will be to be able to take the staircase instead of the elevators for 4 floors if I happen to reach a biological age of 75 years. I want to keep meeting people from varied fields and interests. I want to enhance my interest in music by learning to play the flute.

CLOSING REMARKS

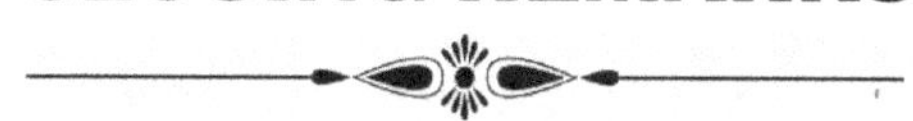

Know yourself. You have to be your first port of call. No one can know you more intimately than yourself.

Find your passion. Anything you are passionate about will not require any motivation.

Be patient with yourself. It takes time to achieve anything. If you have damaged something, it's going to take some time to reverse that damage.

First, acknowledge. Then plan. Then act. Then don't stop. People usually spend too much time planning with little or no action.

Protect your consciousness from hacking. It's being attempted all the time. If you don't guard against it, be assured that it's already being hacked.

Don't search for social validations. It doesn't help. The only person you need validation from is the one reading this sentence.

Surround yourself with people who share similar goals.

Have childlike energy. There is an inner child who has infinite reservoirs of energy. You just need to get in touch with that child.

Avoid multitasking. Humans are Superbad at this. It's a scientific fact.

Never have guilt around food. Change behaviour.

Connect with nature. You are an expression of nature. Bring down the walls of separation between yourself and nature.

Don't mix friendships with business or work.

Cultivate hobbies.

Extract pleasure out of seemingly mundane and routine tasks. They have to be done regardless. Might as well enjoy doing them.

Reverse hack social media. Use it to gain knowledge but on your terms, not by being a prisoner to the artificial intelligence algorithms working in the background.

Set small achievable goals. Many small goals add up to real massive results.

Be inspired but don't mimic.

If it sounds too good- most likely its a consciousness hack.

Believe in possibilities. Things happen.

The distance between you and your goal is - your want.

Your success or failure is in your head. You have to first believe that you can achieve it. Rest is merely rolling out of the act. The script is there in the head.

If you want to achieve something only for yourself-most likely, you will succeed.

Don't be afraid to ask for help. It only shows that you are realistic. There is no ego in seeking help.

Travel and see new places. It's the only life you get to experience the beauty of creation.

There is something inside you which constructs the like's of Mandela, Gandhi, Bolt, Federer, Gates, Bezos. You have to connect to that.

Get into the habit of making notes of even small things. Some of the best ideas were small ideas to start with.

www.ingramcontent.com/pod-product-compliance
Lightning Source LLC
LaVergne TN
LVHW010501200726
843506LV00013B/2484